Never Enough

Never Enough

✦ ✦ ✦ ✦ ✦ ✦

*The Neuroscience and
Experience of Addiction*

Judith Grisel

DOUBLEDAY

NEW YORK

All rights reserved. Published in the United States by Doubleday, a division of Penguin Random House LLC, New York, and distributed in Canada by Random House of Canada, a division of Penguin Random House Canada Limited, Toronto.

www.doubleday.com

DOUBLEDAY and the portrayal of an anchor with a dolphin are registered trademarks of Penguin Random House LLC.

Illustration credits: All line artwork copyright © Lena Miskulin; (Page 55): "CB_1receptors" by Miles Herkenham, National Institute of Mental Health, NIH; (Page 59): "Downregulation of CB_1" by Victoria S. Dalton and Katerina Zavitsanou, from "Cannabinoid Effect on CB_1 Receptor Density in the Adolescent Brain: An Autoradiographic Study Using the Synthetic Cannabinoid HU 210," *Synapse* 64, Issue 11 (March 29, 2010). Copyright © 2010 by Wiley-Liss, Inc. Reprinted by permission of Wiley; (Page 93): "The heritable differences in endorphin signaling" adapted from data published by Gianoulakis et al., from "Different Pituitary Beta-Endorphin and Adrenal Cortisol Response to Ethanol in Individuals with High and Low Risk for Future Development of Alcoholism," *Life Sciences* 45, issue 12 (1989); (Page 141): "MDMA neurotoxicity" by Dr. George Ricarte, Johns Hopkins University School of Medicine.

Jacket design by Emily Mahon

LIBRARY OF CONGRESS CATALOGING-IN-PUBLICATION DATA
Names: Grisel, Judith, author.
Title: Never enough : the neuroscience and experience of addiction / Judith Grisel.
Description: First edition. | New York : Doubleday, [2019] | Includes bibliographical references and index.
Identifiers: LCCN 2018038404 | ISBN 9780385542845 (hardcover alk. paper) | ISBN 9780385542852 (ebook)
Subjects: LCSH: Drug addiction—Psychological aspects. | Substance abuse—Psychological aspects.
Classification: LCC RC564 .G75 2019 | DDC 362.29—dc23
LC record available at https://lccn.loc.gov/2018038404

MANUFACTURED IN THE UNITED STATES OF AMERICA

First Edition

To Marty Devereaux,

without whose love and acceptance

I'd have been unlikely to make it through

either my addiction or my education

Contents

Never Enough

Introduction

I was twenty-two. I'd been on the good end of a bad drug deal. In the wee hours of some morning late in 1985, behind a nameless restaurant in South Florida, a dealer gave me and a friend the wrong bag. I was the "winner" in this deal with substantially more drug than I was obliged to pass on to a friend of a friend somewhere in the Midwest.

Homeless at the time, my compatriot and I ended up checking into a cheap motel in Deerfield Beach. Predictably, we used the surplus along with what we owed. Toward the end of that binge, the stash mercifully depleted, both of us exhausted and on edge, my friend inexplicably announced that there would never be enough cocaine for us. While the prophecy struck me as true even in my overwhelmed state, I also knew it was irrelevant. As with every addict, my days of actually getting "high" were long past. My using was compulsive and aimed more at escaping reality than at getting off. I'd banged my head against the wall long enough to realize that nothing new was going to happen—except perhaps through the ultimate escape, death, which frankly didn't seem like that big a deal.

About six months later, through a series of circumstances rather than personal insight or strength of character, I was clean and sober for the first time in years, and therefore not quite so numb. I saw that I had a life-or-death choice. I could continue colluding with my mental illness as it inexorably consumed me, or I could find a different way to live.

In my experience, very few faced with those possibilities choose life, and I first went with the majority. The cost of abstinence seemed too high: Without drugs, what would there be to live for anyway? However, in a demonstration of tenacity almost diagnostic of an active addict, it dawned on me that I might be able to find another way. After all, I thought, I'd come through many tight situations: bad deals in condemned buildings or police stations, with or without loaded guns, and miles from anything friendly or familiar. Aware now for the first time of the medical model of addiction, I figured that my disease was a biological problem that could be solved. I decided to cure addiction so I could somehow eliminate the problems caused by using.

With what may seem like exceptional fortitude to some, especially given that I'd been kicked out of three schools by this time, I went on to get a Ph.D. in behavioral neuroscience and to become an expert in the neurobiology, chemistry, and genetics of addictive behavior. This accomplishment would seem almost unremarkable to most addicts, who know firsthand that there is nothing we would not do, no sacrifice too great, to be able to use. It ultimately took seven years to graduate from college, including about a year of dramatic change starting in a treatment center, plus another seven years of graduate school to earn that degree.

This book is a summary of what I have learned over the past twenty or so years as a researcher studying the neuroscience of addiction. Though I've received grants from the National Institutes of Health and possess a controlled-substance license from the Drug Enforcement Administration (DEA), I regret to say that I haven't solved the problem. I have, however, learned a lot about how people like me differ even before they pick up their first drug and about what addictive substances do to our brains. My hope is that sharing this information might help loved ones, caregivers, and crafters of public policy make more informed choices. Perhaps this understanding may even help the afflicted ones themselves, because it's quite clear to me that the solution isn't coming in a pill.

+

Addiction today is epidemic and catastrophic. If we are not victims ourselves, we all know someone struggling with a merciless compulsion to remodel experience by altering brain function. The personal and social consequences of this widespread and relentless urge are almost too large to grasp. In the United States, about 16 percent of the population twelve and older meet criteria for a substance use disorder, and about a quarter of all deaths are attributed to excessive drug use. Each day, ten thousand people around the globe die as a result of substance abuse. Along this path to the grave is a breathtaking series of losses: of hope, dignity, relationships, money, generativity, family and societal structure, and community resources.

Worldwide, addiction may be *the* most formidable health problem, affecting about one in every five people over the age of fourteen. In purely financial terms, it costs more than five times as much as AIDS and twice as much as cancer. In the United States, this means that close to 10 percent of all health-care expenditures go toward prevention, diagnosis, and treatment of people suffering from addictive diseases, and the statistics are similarly frightening in most other Western cultures. Despite all this money and effort, successful recovery is no more likely than it was fifty years ago.

There are two primary reasons for the incredibly broad, deep, and persistent costs of drug addiction. First, excessive use is remarkably common, cutting across geographic, economic, ethnic, and gender lines with little variation. It is also highly resistant to treatment. Although reliable estimates are hard to come by, most experts agree that no more than 10 percent of substance abusers can manage to stay clean for any appreciable time. As far as illnesses go, this rate is almost singularly low: one has about twice as good a chance of surviving brain cancer.

Despite a statistically bleak outlook, there are some reasons to be encouraged. Some addicts, once desperate cases, do get clean and stay clean, and even go on to live productive, happy lives. While neuroscience hasn't been able to thoroughly parse the mechanisms behind this transformation, we have learned quite a lot about the causes of the problem. We know, for instance, that addiction results from a complex web of factors including a genetic predisposition, developmental influences, and environmental input. I say complex because each of these factors is very dense. That is, hundreds of genes and innumerable environmental contributions are involved. The factors also depend on one another. For example, a particular strand of DNA may enhance a liability for addiction but only in the presence (or absence) of other specific genes and along with certain experiences during development (either pre- or postnatal) and in specific contexts. So, while we may know a lot, the complexity of the disease means that we are still unable to predict whether a particular individual will develop an addiction.

While in the end there might be as many different paths to addiction as there are addicts, there are general principles of brain function that underlie all compulsive use. My aim in writing this book is to share these principles and thus shed light on the biological dead end that perpetuates substance use and abuse: namely, that there will never be enough drug, because the brain's capacity to learn and adapt is basically infinite. What was once a normal state punctuated by periods of high, inexorably transforms to a state of desperation that is only temporarily subdued by drug. Understanding the mechanisms behind every addict's experience makes it very clear that short of death or long-term sobriety there is no way to quell the screaming need between exposures. At the point where pathology determines behavior, most addicts die trying to satisfy an insatiable drive.

My Story

The first time I got drunk, at thirteen, I felt as Eve should have after tasting the apple. Or as a bird hatched in a cage would feel upon being unexpectedly set free. The drug provided physical relief and spiritual antidote for the persistent restlessness I'd been unable to identify or share. An abrupt shift of perspective coincident with guzzling half a gallon of wine in my friend's basement somehow made me feel sure that both life and I were going to be all right. Just as light is revealed by darkness, and joy by sorrow, alcohol provided powerful subconscious recognition of my desperate strivings for self-acceptance and existential purpose and my inability to negotiate a complex world of relationships, fears, and hopes. At the same time, it seemed to deliver, on a satin pillow, the key to all my blooming angst. Abruptly relieved from an existence both harsh and lackluster, I had finally discovered ease.

Or perhaps that ease was more akin to anesthesia, but at the time and for several years after I not only couldn't tell the difference but didn't care. Until the moment alcohol first filled my belly and brain, I hadn't consciously recognized that I'd been just enduring, but that evening, as I leaned out the open window of my friend's bedroom, gazing at the stars, I took what felt like my first truly deep breaths. A plaque I later saw posted behind a bar described my first experience precisely: "Alcohol makes you feel like you're supposed to feel when you're not drinking alcohol." Among other things, I wondered why, if the drug can do this, didn't everyone drink more, and more often?

So I began with enthusiasm, even determination. From the start, I consumed as much and as often as I could—literally through most of seventh grade, because school afforded the best opportunities for freedom from parental oversight in my suburban, middle-class world. Drinking before, during, and (when I could) after school, I seemed to possess an admirable innate tolerance. I was almost never sick or hungover—perhaps it was my youthful liver—and appeared presentable despite what would surely be deemed legal intoxication. Though I never achieved the overwhelming sense of wholeness that I experienced the first time, alcohol continued to confer muted contentment. Any altered state seemed a dramatic improvement over a drab and tedious life toeing the line.

As far back as I can remember, I felt hemmed in, frustrated by imposed limits and my own limitations. Longing for other, for something else, is at the core of my experience of self. Even today, below the persona of nurturing friend, committed partner, determined scientist, and adoring parent is a heartbreaking desire to embrace oblivion. From what or to where I seek escape, I really can't say; I just know that the constraints of space, time, circumstances, obligations, choices (and missed opportunities) fill me with an overwhelming sense of desperation. In fact, my modal thought is that I'm squandering time, though I am quick to admit that I have no idea what to do with myself. Like in a dream, time flows by as I futilely pursue a series of inane tasks, all the while suppressing a growing sense of panic. I fantasize about disembarking at an unfamiliar exit, or pushing aside a broken gate into a foreign sanctum, somehow entering a world where we all at least agree not to pretend things are different than they seem.

What is going on? What am I doing? Questions like these must have been among my first conscious thoughts. If I tried to speak them to anyone, I'm sure what I heard back were directives to "be good," "work hard," "smile," and "don't get caught." If others didn't share my horror, or at least consternation, I couldn't understand why not, because we were all subject to the same capricious laws of existence, the same evidence for irrational forces. If they did share it, I was amazed and repulsed by their willingness nonetheless to fritter away their lives acquiring things, planning parties, cleaning up, and checking the "news."

Countless people have grappled with feelings of emptiness and despair, but I didn't know that then, and other than a few curious pieces of fiction or poetry, I don't recall a single acknowledgment of bewilderment in those around me until I was well into my teens. My first time getting drunk seemed to offer an easy way through the difficulty of growing up, and it was a long while before I had enough awareness to look back and wonder about the causes of my trajectory. In the end, the very effect I loved so much about alcohol—its ability to mute existential fears—utterly betrayed me. It didn't take all that long before the drug's most reliable effect was to ensure the alienation, despair, and emptiness that I sought to medicate.

The chief of the National Institute on Alcohol Abuse and Alcoholism, George Koob, has said that there are two ways of becoming an alcoholic: either being born one or drinking a lot. Dr. Koob is not trying to be flip, and the high likelihood that one or the other of these applies to each of us helps explain why the disease is so prevalent. I agree that many who end up like me have a predisposition even before their first sip but also appreciate that enough exposure to any mind-altering drug will induce tolerance and dependence—hallmarks of addiction—in anyone with a nervous system. Unfortunately, though, no scientific model can yet explain my quick and brutal slide to homelessness, hopelessness, and utter desolation.

Choosing Oblivion

The next ten years were characterized by a simple philosophy and practice: I sought any opportunity to use mind-altering drugs and paid any cost. My actions only made sense in terms of that guiding principle; virtually every moment was shaped by an orientation toward escaping sober awareness. If my first good drink gave me a sense of peace, the first time I got high was plain fun. Alcohol made life bearable, but weed made it hilarious! And coke made it "hot," and meth, exciting, and acid, interesting . . . For all this pharmacological conjuring, I traded myself away a piece at a time. Many of the experiences I had during this formative time are completely lost to memory, but of those I can recall, some were amusing or fantastic, like the evening just before final exams when I initiated a road trip from St. Louis to Nashville. Others were embarrassing or dangerous, like navigating my grandparents' Suburban with my head out the window because the streetlight seemed so much more informative than the dash or road signage, while several friends clung to the roof, all of us tripping; or climbing into a stranger's speedboat in Miami because I was bored with my date. But the majority are painful.

I ended up attending college at a Jesuit school in the heartland, despite fancying myself at a state school in California, because my mother filled out my college applications. Though I had some excellent teachers and did okay my first semester, it didn't take long to find my kind. By early in my second term, I had a fake ID and knew where to score pot, able to pick up right where I left off after graduating from high school high as a kite in South Florida. I'm sure I'm not the only person for whom college was an opportunity to get out from under a watchful parental glare, and the freedom to do what I wanted was exhilarating. I spent most of my time drinking and partying and only studied or went to class as a last resort.

Where did all this freedom lead? I have a clear memory of lying in my bunk one afternoon, stoned but despairing. Students were chatting as they walked outside my window or down the hall; I had assignments due or overdue and probably plans to meet up with friends for dinner. However, I was overwhelmed by a sense of emptiness and futility even more intense than usual. I can't think of anything in my circumstances that precipitated this crisis; even now I think of my drug use—especially in the early stages—as much cure as cause. But for whatever reason, I saw my whole life, despite blips of disaster and achievement, as an aimless trajectory of self-preservation and promotion: starting and going nowhere, and characterized by reflexive and blind occupation. Moreover, it seemed that my life was no different from anyone else's. We were like fish schooling in circles, oblivious to the water and indifferent to anything outside our own self-serving heads. I remember the gray and formless pit in my chest and belly that these thoughts evoked. Each of us was completely alone, and our efforts were primarily directed at maintaining delusions that kept us sane, until we died.

The only rational response, I thought, was to kill myself, but the aesthetic of the whole thing struck me as pathetic. Despite thinking all was vanity, I was still quite vain, and leaping from my dorm window just didn't feel like my style. Instead, that afternoon represented a turning point in my addiction. An avid user from the start, I now was truly committed. My behavior became reckless and spiraled quickly toward a life that matched my ideas of existence in terms of heartless insanity.

In other words, my response to being overwhelmed by the

deep void was to leap into it. I'd traipse back from bars in East St. Louis, alone, drunk and stoned, in the early hours of the morning. Several weeks were spent in a housing project with a group of locals I had nothing in common with except an appreciation for freebase cocaine (this, in the days just before crack), while "their" women and children hung out in a windowless bedroom watching TV. I'd end up in an assortment of sordid places completely unprepared and thought testing my wit against whoever or whatever happened to be in my face was a somewhat less tedious way to pass the time as I entertained death.

The school decided I should take a break at the same time my parents realized they were being taken. I remember the day, standing in our driveway, when they announced they were withdrawing financial support. I wish I could say I felt sorry, especially as my little brother, a brawny high school football player, bawled in the street, but in fact all I remember is exhilaration. No more limits! No more having to please and satisfy authority! A girlfriend who in important ways was like a twin picked me up, and we checked into a Howard Johnson's after pooling our money to buy a blender, juice, and two gallons of vodka. My first taste of adulthood was off to a fine start.

For the next three years or so, I lived and worked here and there, often scraping by on nothing but lies and evasion. The only constant was using. Whether with or without a job, a home, or other conventional resources, I always managed to find a way to get (and more or less stay) loaded. Before being fired for skimming the till, I worked at a classless bar on the railroad tracks called Tips Tavern. Regulars arrived with their paychecks on Friday afternoon to pay off their tabs and were usually starting new ones before the end of the night. My parents really detached, and I rarely saw family. I vaguely remember a grandparent's funeral where I was wasted on quaaludes and struggled to contrive an appropriate countenance while I felt absolutely nothing. It was much later, after some time substance-free, that I was able to mourn anything, including the loss of my grandfather.

Another time I was mid-inhale on a fat roach, holding it to my mouth at a stoplight, when I looked to my left and saw both my parents, their hands frozen in a wave. I remember the bright day, and the joy turned sadness in their faces as all three of us looked away quickly. I might have thought how unlikely it was that we all happened to be at the same intersection, but actually it wasn't that big of a town, and the truth is, I *never* got in a car without at least a joint and a couple of beers or a mixed drink. I was flooded in shame for just a bit longer than it took me to alter my course and take another hit. Today I look back on my compulsive self with as much compassion as I feel for my parents.

Until about ten seconds before the first time I used a needle, I thought I'd never inject drugs. Like most people, I associated needles with hard-core use. That is, until I was offered a shot. I remember feeling for an instant before acquiescing as if I really could choose; I didn't recognize crossing this line as inevitable, as it would be the second through nth time, but rather felt as if I would just like to try it. I tasted and heard the coke before I felt it: an unusual tang on the back of my tongue coupled by ringing in my ears like a fire alarm. Then I felt it! A warm wash of euphoria that was so much richer than that from snorting as my body and brain grew warm and wet and interested, and I felt gratitude for the brilliance of living. I'm not exaggerating when I say that a few minutes later I was in charge of the point, in part so I could be sure my turn wasn't skipped. Still more than a long year away, administering cocaine in this way, precipitated my early bottom.

Though I ripped off stores and stole credit cards when the

opportunity presented itself, I was still able to maintain, at least to myself, that I was basically a good person. To an extent, for instance, I could count on my companions, and they could count on me. I say to an extent, because we also knew and expected that we would lie, cheat, or steal from each other if something really important were at stake (that is, drugs). For instance, when we'd pool our money to score, it was best if we all went to the pickup together. On occasions where just one, or a subset, would go, it was pretty much understood that the bag would be a little lighter by the time it arrived. No one should be expected to be that trustworthy! However, I remember one incident when a boyfriend and I planned to go to a neighboring town to watch Fourth of July fireworks. Some guy we knew, an acquaintance from work maybe, didn't have plans, and so we invited him along. At the time, I felt generous because he was all alone and a little bit sad, and we were nice enough to let him share our evening. We drank and smoked our way through the festivities, and the next day I found a wad of bills in the back of the car. Three hundred dollars. My boyfriend and I discussed it and decided to keep the money. I knew this was unethical, even by my lax standards, in part because it was so hard to justify; something about how we'd helped him out and needed to pay our rent. Later, when he asked, I looked the unsuspecting friend right in his eyes and said, "No, I haven't seen it . . . bum luck." I knew he needed the cash and that what I had done and said was simply wrong. We ended up buying an eight ball with the money.

Another story: Johnny was a Vietnam vet who lived next door in a crappy apartment behind the high school. A gentle and hopeless guy, he was lonely enough to share his drugs. Johnny's life dream was to be maintained in a hospital bed with a permanent line for IV drug infusions. Under different circumstances, he might have been a friend, but friendship depends on trust and supporting each other's well-being. One day we were slamming coke in his filthy room, when his eyes rolled back and he fell down convulsing. I stepped out of the way and thought, "He probably won't want his next bump." He didn't die that day, but of the three of us in the room I'm the only one still alive.

I share these stories not to make readers uncomfortable (and I'm sorry if they do) or solely to qualify myself as a bona fide addict. My primary purpose in exposing my story is to illustrate the depths, as well as the breadth (in later chapters), of the addictive experience. I don't think I was basically a good person who got mixed up with a bad crowd, for instance, or that I was somehow dealt a crummy hand in terms of genes or neurochemistry, parents, or personal history (though these all certainly had an influence). I also don't think that I am essentially worse than or even different from others: not those spending down their allotment of days under bridges, or in prisons, or for that matter managing PTAs or running for public office. All of us face countless choices, and there is no bright line separating good and bad, order and entropy, life and death. Perhaps as a result of following rules or conventions, some live under the delusion that they are innocent, safe, or deserving of their status as well-fed citizens. But if there is a devil, it lives inside each of us. One of my greatest assets is knowing that my primary enemy is not outside me, and for this I am grateful to all my experiences. We all have the capacity for wrong; otherwise we could not, in fact, be free.

The opposite of addiction, I have learned, is not sobriety but choice. For many like me, drugs act as potent tools that obscure freedom. But there are countless ways any of us might jump the rail, unwrapping familiar cloaks of vocation, family, or other disguise. As James Baldwin put it, "Freedom is hard to bear"; for those who don't recognize the tenuousness of the situation, just pray that habits, bank accounts, or other props remain securely in place.

Bearing Change

They say that every recovery is birthed at the bottom. For my part, it's a miracle I didn't get what I deserved, and being sure of this is much better than thinking I deserve more than I've gotten. The start of the end was kicked off behind that unremarkable restaurant on Route 1, where the dealer handed over the wrong bag and my friend offered his surprising insight that there would simply never be enough cocaine.

This must have struck a deep chord, because the echo of Steve's words has been rolling like a marble down a culvert ever since. Lines connecting dots are hazy, but that jag constituted my last big coke binge. As a result, in addition to just barely escaping the AIDS virus, I was able to get a little ahead financially and ended up pooling resources with a couple of friends to pay first and last on a one-bedroom apartment. This provided some advantages to living under bridges or piers, including having privacy to hide piles of empties and other evidence of debauchery. The apartment also had a fridge, usually with electricity, facilitating an easier and more effective way to keep beer cold, and hence a switch from 40s to cases. Finally, of course, there was a bathroom: the propitious site for the bottom of my bottom. Though not much for primping, one day just after getting up (and therefore at the nadir of my internal pharmacopoeia), I had a terrifying encounter—with myself. About three inches from the mirror, I was peering into my own eyes and was met with a clear vision of the bottomless abyss inside me. I felt as though I were looking into my own soul and what I confronted was worse than the emptiness I'd been running from, much worse.

My response, naturally, was to head straight for the bong, but still I couldn't shake the creeped-out feeling that day, or for a long while after. I felt haunted by a truth so lorn it made my strategies for evasion look like decorations at the gallows. I think of the moment in the mirror as my bottom because it was probably the closest I'd come to seeing myself in many years, and though what I saw might not have been all of me, it was enough to destroy many of my illusions. For the following three or so months, I was incapable of consuming enough of anything to blot out that image.

The dam was finally breached during a visit with my father. I was surprised when he offered to take me to dinner for my twenty-third birthday, because we hadn't spoken in years. Family ties are deep, though, and below all of my self-righteous anger, I still wanted his love and approval, so when he made the offer, I readily accepted.

The day we were to go out, my main concern was to manage my dosing so as to shelter my interactions with him and still remain upright. This was a legitimate worry. By this time, I had almost no relationships that involved expectations, and I knew it was impossible to sleep anything off before an "early bird" dinner, especially because I woke most days after noon. I literally had no idea what to do with four to five hours of free time if I wasn't getting wasted. At any rate, I was only a bit toasty when I climbed into his car, and vainly hoping not obviously so. We arrived at the restaurant, which had been my choice, a tiny sushi place with a few small tables and the requisite bar, a few minutes later. I didn't feel particularly vulnerable and also wasn't expecting much. So I was completely caught off guard when my father strangely announced that he just wanted me to be happy. This may possibly be the very last thing I expected to hear; he might have wished me to go back to school, sit up straight, repay what I owed, or take better care of my teeth. But be happy?

Where did this father come from? (To this day, he can't recall the conversation, and no one's heard him say anything this out of character since.) But my *dad* saying he wished me to *be happy* somehow collapsed my defenses, and I was suddenly blubbering into my miso about how incredibly miserable I was! Despite arranging things to my own liking, by eliminating limits and responsibilities and partying nonstop—I was entirely discontented. So much so that despite extensive experience flaunting bravado, I couldn't muster even a modicum of my usual arrogance as he, along with the other patrons, the waitstaff, and probably even the cook, witnessed my sloppy undoing.

When I first arrived for treatment, I lacked both understanding and acceptance. I had no idea what I'd signed on for (unbelievably, I had been envisioning a spa), just jumped at the chance for escape, as always. Adulthood is characterized more than anything else by a capacity to see beyond one's own narrow perspective, and an intake evaluation by the treatment center suggested I'd be best suited for the children's program; I have no doubt they were right on. It was fortunate my parents brought me all the way to Minnesota. If I'd been anywhere near anything or anyone I knew, I'd surely have gone AWOL rather than face the many ways I'd been colluding in my own ruin. Instead, I stayed at the treatment center for twenty-eight days and then spent three months in a women's halfway house, aptly named Progress Valley. Talk about a stark introduction to reality: this was a former convent on the side of an interstate filled with infantile brats like me, with rules concerning everything from naps to tea saucers.

However, it was there that I began to realize that my initial intuitions about alcohol and other drugs were precisely upside down. Rather than provide a solution to my problems with living, they had chipped away at every prospect until only the barest shred of life remained. I'd sought wellness and became sick; fun, but lived in a constant state of anxious dread; freedom, and was enslaved. In just ten years, my sources for solace had totally betrayed me, carving out a canyon deep and unlivable. Drugs were destroying every aspect of my life, yet my days revolved around self-administering until I passed out.

By the time I turned twenty-three, it had been years since I'd gone even twenty-four hours without a drink, pill, fix, or joint. Though the fun and excitement were long gone, I also could not wrap my head around having a disease that necessitated a lifetime of abstinence. I know now that the drugs were still dispensing a mite of escape, and therefore offered a more appealing option than exposing myself raw and unmedicated to the elements of living. But dying slowly a day at a time was turning out to be unbearably painful. I'd finally reached the dead end where I felt I was incapable of living either with or without mind-altering substances. This bleak situation describes the condition of many, if not all, addicts and illustrates why relatively few recover. Despite being depleted, they think the cost of abstinence seems much too high: Without drugs, what is there to live for anyway?

Eventually, two factors motivated my desire to recover. First, I began to wonder just a wee bit about what it would be like to live in the relatively uncharted territory of sobriety. I'd been scraping around the basement floor for so long it seemed as if it might at least be interesting to explore another place. I thought of myself as courageous (facing lunatic dealers and DEA agents with aplomb), and it was equal parts courage and curiosity that contributed to the decision to give abstinence a try. I promised myself that if I wasn't less miserable sober than I'd been loaded, I'd go back to using. Because I had some notion that such a change in lifestyle would suck for a while, my plan included a specific date for reassessment. In true form, I made sure of a back door.

My second motivation was a decision to find a cure. The arrogance of this astounds me now. But I also think that some of the traits that facilitated my addiction have helped to make me a good scientist. Bottomless curiosity, a willingness to take risks, and perseverance that make a bulldog seem laid-back have all contributed to the successes I've had as a neuroscientist.

More than anything else, seeking and acquiring knowledge about drugs, addiction, and the brain have given me compassion for the desperate plight of people like me. The understanding I've gained has helped me stay clean by informing better choices. My hope is that by illuminating the seeming insanity of colluding in habits that are not only joyless but lethal, this book will contribute to a path of freedom for others.

1

Brain Food

> Never does nature say one thing and
> wisdom another.
>
> —Juvenal (Roman poet, A.D. 60–130)

Why, if I wanted to cure addiction, did I set out to become a neuroscientist, rather than a medical doctor, psychotherapist, or even a self-help guru? Like many others at the time, I believed that the few pounds of fatty goop inside my skull were ultimately responsible for the totality of my condition. Medical and social interventions, if they worked at all, would have to do so via their influence on brain functioning. Therefore, it seemed most straightforward and efficient to focus my efforts on understanding the neural mechanisms behind the states that seemed to define my experience, such as impulsivity and craving. I thought that if I could find the cellular switch that flipped somewhere between my third and my fourth drinks, or each time a promising bag was in my sight, and then find a way to keep this switch in the "off" position, I might be able to refrain from telling off the few people with whom I was still on speaking terms, or spending all my tips on very temporary thrills, or making blacked-out road trips to Dallas. In other words, I'd be able to use "like a lady." The idea that *I am my brain* still guides the efforts of thousands of neuroscientists around the world as we work to connect experience to neural structures, chemical interactions, and genes.

Though plausible, I should mention that an elegant hypothesis is no substitute for definitive data. As time has passed, we have learned that everything from the bacteria in our guts to the interactions we had in middle school partly determines our behavior. In fact, it's beginning to seem that the brain is more like a stage for our life to be acted out upon than like the director behind a curtain calling shots. Nonetheless, it's reasonable to assume that all of our thoughts, feelings, intentions, and behaviors at least have *correlates* in electrical and chemical signals in the brain, because there's not a whit of evidence to suggest otherwise.

Though the central nervous system (CNS)—that is, the brain and the spinal cord—is mind-bogglingly complex, it is not oversimplifying to say that its cells are continuously occupied with two principal tasks: responding to the environment and then adapting to it. These two basic functions are key to understanding how drugs work and how addiction develops. We'll spend this chapter covering how drugs produce their effects in the brain and the next one on how the brain adapts to those influences and, in doing so, creates addiction.

The CNS is our sole means of interacting with the environment. Most neural real estate is employed in sensing, perceiving, and reacting to what is around us. Many good thinkers, from philosophers to novelists, have speculated about who we would be without access to the environment. Aren't our intentions, feelings, and activities all stimulus-driven, at least to some extent? The classic antiwar novel *Johnny Got His Gun*[1] raises questions about what life would be like if we were unable to sense or respond to the world around us. After nearly being killed in battle, the protagonist wakes in a hospital bed, only to realize that his limbs and face are gone and that he cannot move, speak, see, hear, or smell. The story takes place over several years as Joe grapples with profound limitations—wondering, for instance, how to tell waking from sleeping in the absence of interactions with the environment.

Though Joe's plight is surely the stuff of nightmares, it's not as though any of us accurately experiences what is around us. Far from it! For instance, many insects can see ultraviolet light that for us is, literally, invisible. Similarly, we cannot detect vibrations in air molecules of very high or low frequency (as bats or elephants readily perceive), which means we can't hear very high- or low-pitched sounds, even though they too are all around us. And while we may see better than dogs—who happen to smell about a thousand times better than we do—a typical pigeon has much better eyesight than humans do. So, we are all prisoners of our nervous system to some extent. Even within a species, there are differences in sensitivity, and a single individual may demonstrate significant variation across his or her lifetime. For instance, women can typically detect higher-pitched sounds than men, but we all become less sensitive to these as we age. And the vast majority of us are trichromats, meaning that we perceive thousands of different colors by the combined activity in just three types of color-sensitive neurons. But some lucky individuals have a mutation that gives them a fourth type of color sensor, and even though they may not be aware of their mutant gift, they are more likely to have careers as artists or designers. The most important lesson here, though, is that our senses constrain our experience by offering us a relatively thin slice of what's out there—a highly filtered version of our environment.

Part of the CNS's genius is its ability to convert environmental signals into its native vocabulary of electrical and chemical energy. To say that all abused drugs are sensed by the nervous system is to say that they all reliably alter this electrical and chemical brain activity, just as a pebble tossed into a pond produces discernible ripples. When I was just beginning my experimental drug use as a teen, there was a popular TV public-service announcement with the refrain "This is your brain on drugs," showing an egg dropped into a frying pan, where it sizzled and cooked—implying that drugs were like embalming fluid for the brain. Although it might have captured attention, the argument was entirely vacuous, and even a ninth grader's level of critical thinking skills could see right through it. Every single thing we experience—including drugs certainly, but also propaganda, walks in the woods, lunch with friends, falling in love, making or not making the point/sale/grade—is registered as structural and functional changes on the frying pan of our brain, which is precisely why they are experiences. Here's your brain on skiing . . . on daydreaming . . . on anger . . . on fear. The brain is no more static than a river as currents constantly form from the flow of our experience. In this way, and in others, we are shaped by our environment.

So, in order for us to experience anything at all, our nervous system must be altered by the experience. This reality of constant change spawns a paradox, which is that those changes can only be perceived against a background of neural stability.

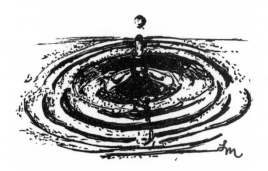

Because we encounter an ever-variable environment as we go about our day, if our neural activity simply reflected all of this input, like the ocean in the midst of a storm, then the tossed pebble, or even a boulder, could have no perceptible impact. In neuro-parlance, the ratio of signal to noise would be too low. In order for a stimulus to be detected, let alone interpreted as meaningful, the neural signal must be greater than the background noise—or the noise must be quashed.

The fundamental role of the brain is to be a contrast detector. As experiences are distinguished from monotony, they spark neurochemical changes in specific brain circuits, informing us of all we care to know: opportunities for food, drink, or sex; danger or pain; beauty and pleasure, for example. The process of actively maintaining the stable baseline critical for conducting the brain's business of contrast detection is called homeostasis, and it depends on having a set point, a comparator, and a mechanism for adjustment. It is easy to appreciate this principle in terms of body temperature, which is maintained around ninety-nine degrees Fahrenheit. If you become much warmer or colder than this, your body feels it, and there are mechanisms to return you to baseline, such as sweating or shivering. Feelings are also constrained within tight bounds under normal conditions. What we generally experience is our personal neutral okayness; otherwise we'd be incapable of detecting "good" or "bad" events.

We'll return to homeostasis later. For now we'll consider what makes abused drugs remarkable—their ability to hijack the contrast detector for pleasure.

Wired for News

In the 1950s, two Canadian researchers conducted an experiment typical of the period.[2] Under general anesthesia they implanted an electrode (a thin wire that conducts electricity) into a rat's brain, in the location of a specific neural circuit. After the rat fully recovered, they sent mild electric currents through the electrode to mimic natural activity in order to study the effects on the rat's behavior and identify the circuit's function.

At first James Olds and Peter Milner thought they had discovered the cells responsible for curiosity, because the rat in their experiment kept returning to the area of its cage that had been paired with the electric current. After continued experimentation, however, the researchers concluded that they had found a site for pleasure, and they called it the brain's "reward center." In subsequent experiments, when a rat was given the ability to press a bar to stimulate this region of its own brain, it did so with abandon and to the exclusion of virtually everything else. For example, a hungry rat would ignore food to turn on the electrical current, and males occupied with turning on the current disregarded sexually receptive females (a stimulus usually more powerful than food). In some cases, their single-minded quest to stimulate this area of the brain resulted in starvation and sleep deprivation to the point of death.

The parallel to drug addiction was immediately obvious. Over ensuing decades, the circuitry identified by Olds and Milner has been the subject of thousands of studies that have helped clarify its anatomic, chemical, and genetic components, as well as its connection to behavior. Most critically, we know that the electrical stimulation they applied led to release of the neurotransmitter dopamine in the nucleus accumbens (a-COME-benz). This is an area of the brain located about three inches behind the bottom of the eye sockets and is part of the limbic system, a group of structures that are primarily involved in emotion. The dopamine was released here by neurons that originate in the midbrain, following the mesolimbic pathway (so called because it goes from the midbrain, that is, *meso,* to the limbic system).

All drugs affect multiple brain circuits, and variation in their sites of neural action accounts for their different effects. However, all addictive drugs are addictive precisely because they share the ability to stimulate the mesolimbic dopamine system. Countless studies have demonstrated that the squirt of dopamine in the nucleus accumbens from addictive substances (including chocolate and hot sauce!) is associated with the substances' pleasurable outcome. Some, like cocaine and amphetamine, are universally effective; others seem to have a bigger influence on mesolimbic dopamine in some individuals than in others (for example, marijuana and alcohol), and some that have been labeled addictive probably aren't. For instance, most research suggests that the psychedelic LSD does not stimulate the mesolimbic pathway. From this and related evidence, the majority of addiction researchers would argue that LSD is not an addictive drug.

Early on, a few depressed patients were implanted with electrodes so that they could self-stimulate the mesolimbic circuit in an attempt to help them feel better. Unfortunately, rather than being cured of depression as their doctors had hoped, these patients just became *really distracted* pressing their own "bars." The clinical trials ended because they were deemed ineffective and perhaps even unethical. The mesolimbic system evolved to promote behaviors such as eating and sex, and the sense of pleasure it confers is not so much a mood state as an emotional experience of "thrill" or pleasure, like that associated with sexual foreplay. We now also understand that the opposite of pleasure is not depression but anhedonia, the inability to experience pleasure. Of course, depression and anhedonia are not mutually exclusive, because many depressed individuals also have difficulty experiencing pleasure. But in general, the mesolimbic pathway conveys a transient good time, not a stable sense of hopefulness that would truly serve as an antidote to depression.

When activity in the mesolimbic pathway is prevented—either physically by severing neurons or pharmacologically with drugs that block dopamine—organisms are unable to experience pleasure. So, if the pathway were somehow lesioned before a shot of alcohol or bump of cocaine, especially if these were among your initial experiences with those substances, you'd think the drugs were a complete waste of money (though you'd be sedated or behaviorally active, depending on which drug you had because those effects are produced elsewhere).

This might look like a cure, but as the doctors in the depression study found, it is ethically problematic. Such an intervention would prevent pleasure from all sources, including things like food and sex. Most of the world has prohibited this sort of surgical intervention, although some nations, including China

Mesolimbic pathway

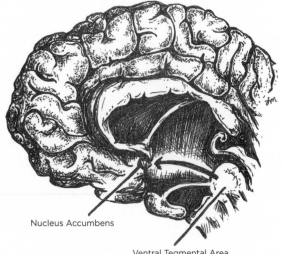

Nucleus Accumbens

Ventral Tegmental Area

and the Soviet Union, are reportedly reducing relapse rates by employing this strategy.[3] However, it doesn't work all that well for seasoned addicts who use mainly to avoid unpleasant symptoms associated with withdrawal rather than seeking a high. Furthermore, generally speaking, even addicts who are clearly suffering in the face of a desperate habit are not willing to voluntarily undergo procedures that produce such a global deficit in joie de vivre. Most would rather go to prison or experience other severe consequences, because at least transient pleasures are still possible. Without dopamine in the nucleus accumbens, nothing, not a letter from a friend, an especially beautiful sunset or piece of music, or even chocolate, would alleviate a persistently bleak existence.

To Groove and to Move

In recent years, new evidence has shown that dopamine in the mesolimbic pathway works not exactly by signaling pleasure but by signaling the *anticipation* of pleasure. This anticipatory state is not the same as the pleasure associated with satisfaction, contentment, or release, but rather the anxious, lip-smacking foretaste of something of import that is just around the corner.

Things that cause a release of dopamine in the mesolimbic pathway may be something pleasurable (sexual stimulation, a bump of cocaine) but also something surprising (drama, whatever is in the package), novel (such as travel), potentially newsworthy (a lottery ticket), or *really* valuable (oxygen to a deprived organism). In other words, this system alerts us to the anticipation of a meaningful event, not to pleasure per se. Pleasurable stimuli happen to be meaningful, but many other things are also inherently meaningful to an organism that has evolved to survive in ever-changing conditions.

There is a second dopamine circuit as well that figures in addiction. Dopamine in the nigrostriatal pathway (which connects the substantia nigra at the base of the brain to the striatum, a large piece of real estate roughly in the center of each hemisphere) enables us to take action either toward or away from a stimulus. As dopamine release in the nucleus accumbens signals something newsworthy happening in the environment, it also activates this second circuit to motivate us to move.

If lesions of the mesolimbic circuit lead to anhedonia, what happens if the nigrostriatal pathway is eliminated? This produces a fairly common condition, especially in the aged. Deficits of dopamine in the nigrostriatal pathway are responsible for Parkinson's disease. Parkinson's sufferers have extreme difficulty enacting their intentions. For instance, people with Parkinson's describe an incredible mental effort required to do a simple motor task such as buttoning a shirt. Parkinsonian deficits occur *between* the desire to move and the movement circuitry, which are both intact.

How does the nigrostriatal lesion in Parkinson's patients occur? Dopamine in both pathways naturally declines with age, partly accounting for general decreases in the eagerness to explore new things and the ability to quickly move toward them. But even before we get old, there are individual differences in dopamine activity, distributed normally, as shown in a bell curve, with those on the low end generally at greater risk for Parkinson's. Besides being slower to enact intentions, low dopamine is also associated with higher-than-average orderliness, conscientiousness, and frugality. In other words, it confers a tendency toward rigidity in areas other than movement.

To sum all this up, dopamine in the mesolimbic circuit leads us to appreciate opening doors, and dopamine in the nigrostriatal circuit enables us to do so. Drugs of abuse (as well as natural

Bell curve

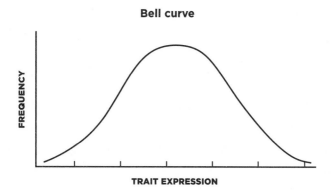

FREQUENCY

TRAIT EXPRESSION

reinforcers like food and sex) stimulate both of these pathways, which is how drugs make us feel good and why we seek them.

Many evolutionarily significant stimuli act as natural reinforcers by stimulating dopamine in both pathways. Some obviously benefit our survival and that of our offspring, like eating and sex, but others are subtler, such as a pleasant social interaction or music (a forerunner of language). Any of these natural incentives pale in comparison to the potency of abused drugs. An obvious reason for the overblown power of drugs is that we control their delivery. Endorphins are natural compounds that stimulate dopamine release and are the basis for effects of opiate drugs. They are synthesized and released in response to a wide range of environmental signals including exercise, sex, sweets, and even stress. In some cases, a natural endorphin surge can be very strong, but it comes nowhere close to the flood from products derived from poppy fields and lab benches and administered by syringe.

Another aspect of our control over delivery is timing. Natural stimuli increase activity of the mesolimbic system by recruiting chemicals in a cascade of neural changes that come about gradually, generally after a few minutes. Drugs, on the other hand, are

absorbed rapidly and act directly to produce nearly instantaneous changes in neurotransmitter levels, including dopamine.
The difference is something like the slow bloom of dawn versus switching on a floodlight. The interval between exposures
to drugs is also unnatural in an evolutionary sense: we decide
when to stop at the package store or the dealer's, so dosing is
more frequent and reliable than for natural stimuli, and likely
much more regular than our evolutionary history provided for.

In general, the more predictable and frequent the dosing, the
more addictive a drug will be.

Three Laws of Psychopharmacology

The very definition of an addictive drug is one that stimulates
the mesolimbic pathway, but there are three general axioms in
psychopharmacology that also apply to all drugs:

1. All drugs act by changing the rate of what is already
   going on.
2. All drugs have side effects.
3. The brain adapts to all drugs that affect it by
   counteracting the drug's effects.

The first law states that drugs can't do anything new, which
is because they only work at all by interacting with existing
brain structures. It follows that drugs can either speed up or
slow down ongoing neural activity—and that's it. Every drug
has a chemical structure (a three-dimensional shape) that is
complementary to certain structures in the brain and produces
its effects by interacting with those structures. For instance,
drugs such as nicotine, delta-9-THC (the active ingredient in
marijuana), and heroin work because they substitute for the

neurotransmitters acetylcholine, anandamide, and endorphin, respectively, interacting at the receptor sites built to interact with those neurotransmitters. Exogenous (made outside the body) drugs often work this way because their shape sufficiently mimics endogenous (made inside the body) neurotransmitters.

The second law is that all drugs have side effects. This is because, unlike normal neurotransmitters, drugs are not targeted in their delivery to precise cells or circuits. Drugs are usually delivered from the blood and found in fairly uniform concentrations throughout the nervous system. They act at all accessible targets, which is to say that they act wherever they encounter a receptive structure. For example, serotonin is a neurotransmitter involved (along with other endogenous chemicals) in many different behaviors such as sleep, aggression, sex, eating, and mood. Serotonin release in the normally functioning brain is targeted to particular cells at particular times, depending on whether it is time to sleep, time to fight, time to eat, and so on. But drugs that enhance or attenuate serotonin act in all these places at once rather than in precise circuits. Therefore, if you take such a drug to modify mood, it will also produce side effects in other motivated behaviors such as sleeping and sex.

The third law is the most interesting of the three axioms, and the one especially relevant to addiction. It concerns the response of the brain to drugs (as opposed to how drugs act on the brain). I'll say much more about this in chapter 2, but for now it is worth noting that the relationship between drugs and the brain is bidirectional. The brain is not just a passive recipient of drug actions but responds to the effects of the drugs. Repeated administration of any drug that influences brain activity leads the brain to adapt in order to *compensate* for the changes associated with the drug.

To illustrate, I consider myself squeaky clean despite a fairly ardent love of coffee. Like most consumers, I drink coffee because I appreciate the arousing effects of caffeine, which acts in the brain by speeding up a part of the nervous system involved in arousal. Before I became a devotee, I suppose I opened my eyes in the morning and felt pretty much awake. It would have taken a few minutes to become fully alert, but my nervous system, entrained to circadian rhythms, would kick in its own arousing mechanisms as an effective way to begin the day. No longer is this the case. I now need coffee to feel normal in the morning, and it would take something like a locomotive coming through the bedroom for me to feel aroused without it. This is because my brain has adapted to the flood of caffeine each morning and has suppressed the natural arousal associated with greeting a new day. Rather than feel normal before coffee and wide awake after, I now feel lethargic before I get it and only begin to approach normalcy with the second cup.

This change in my behavior reflects the states of tolerance (we need more of the drug to achieve its effects) and dependence (without the drug we feel symptoms of withdrawal). The terrible truth for all those who love mind-altering chemicals is that if the chemicals are used with regularity, the brain always adapts to compensate. An addict doesn't drink coffee because she is tired; she is tired because she drinks coffee. Regular drinkers don't have cocktails in order to relax after a rough day; their day is filled with tension and anxiety because they drink so much. Heroin produces euphoria and blocks pain in a naive user, but addicts can't kick a heroin habit, because without it they are in excruciating pain. **The brain's response to a drug is always to facilitate the opposite state; therefore, the only way for any regular user to feel normal is to take the drug.** Getting high, if it occurs at all, is increasingly short-lived, and so the purpose of using is to stave off withdrawal.

This axiom applies to every effect of any drug that results from the drug impacting the brain—including, of course, the release of our old friend dopamine. At first, drugs produce good feelings because molecules of the drug reach the brain, where they impact the nucleus accumbens and other structures to perturb the neutral-okay feeling state. However, the brain, designed to return the system to its homeostatic set point, counteracts the squirts of dopamine interpreted as pleasure or possibility. This consequence turns out to be the driving force and scourge of regular drug users, inspiring the urge to use and then ensuring its perpetuation, because with repeated exposure to the same stimulus over time, there are smaller and smaller changes in dopamine. Eventually, exposure to a favorite drug results in virtually no change in mesolimbic dopamine, but withholding it leads to a big drop, which we experience as a feeling of disappointment and craving. Thus the most profound law of drug use is this: there is no free lunch.

2

Adaptation

> The principal activities of brains
> are making changes in themselves.
>
> —Marvin L. Minsky, 1927–2016 (from
> *The Society of Mind,* 1986)

Brain Change

On the last day of his life, shortly before being forced to drink poison for failing to believe in the state-endorsed gods and for corrupting youth, Socrates engaged in a final dialogue with his students. This teaching, reported by Plato in *Phaedo,* is focused mostly on the nature of the soul but includes a comment about the relationship between pleasure and pain. After a prison guard has removed his chains, Socrates purportedly noted, "How singular is the thing called pleasure, and how curiously related to pain, which might be thought to be the opposite of it . . . he who pursues either of them is generally compelled to take the other. They are two, and yet they grow together out of one head or stem." This philosophical observation, recorded around 350 B.C.E., astutely predicted the experimental insights of the nineteenth-century French physiologist Claude Bernard. Bernard is credited as the first to note that moving between opposite biological states enables our bodies to maintain stability in the face of disruption—anything from a sudden change in the weather to a bad grade on a paper or a death in the family.

Bernard was a single-minded scientist who agreed to an arranged marriage because his wife's dowry provided funding for his early experiments. He'd already published several groundbreaking studies by the mid-1850s, when he came up with a theory that has broad implications for our understanding of physiology and special relevance for addiction. Bernard observed that "the stability of the internal environment [*milieu intérieur*] is the condition for the free and independent life."[1] We face a constant stream of challenges to the *milieu intérieur*, he continued, and he noticed that in each case, at "every instant," we maintain a dynamic equilibrium, essentially a stable *milieu intérieur*, achieved through continuous adjustment.

About eighty years later, an American physiologist, Walter Cannon, who also coined the pithy description "fight or flight," popularized Bernard's ideas in a book titled *The Wisdom of the Body*.[2] In it, he described the tendency toward equilibrium as a function of a process he termed homeostasis. It took another fifty or so years for Richard Solomon, an experimental psychologist working at the University of Pennsylvania, to clarify how homeostasis applies to feelings, and thus to pave the way for our current understanding of addiction.

Working with his student John Corbit, Solomon suggested that any and every stimulus that perturbs the way we feel is actively counteracted by the nervous system in order to return to homeostasis. The stimulus could be a drug but also good or bad news, falling in love, or skydiving. In their opponent-process theory, Solomon and Corbit made the case[3] that feeling states are maintained around a "set point" just as body temperature and water balance are. They proposed that any feeling, including "good," "bad," "happy," "depressed," or "excited," for example, represents a disruption of the stable feeling state that we perceive as "neutral." Specifically, the opponent-process theory posits that **any stimulus that alters brain functioning to affect the way we feel will elicit a response by the brain that is exactly opposite to the effect of the stimulus.** As Newton might succinctly put it: who goes up, must come down.

Say our brain detects an external stimulus that produces either pleasant or unpleasant feelings. According to Solomon and Corbit, in either case the brain responds by counteracting those feelings. For instance, suppose that you have a medical test that indicates cancer. It's very likely, in such a case, that initial feelings of panic or despair give way to a general state of worry as you grapple with myriad implications. These less intense feelings endure while your test results look bad. However, if things change, perhaps a biopsy comes back clear, rather than return to your original state, you would likely experience a period of elation—in effect, a mirror image of the despair you had felt. This pattern of change in affective experience is elicited by any event that pushes the brain beyond its neutral set point.

Though we're usually unaware of affective homeostasis at work, most of us will recognize this pattern in the feeling states surrounding romantic love. It's typical to experience dramatic affective changes as you "fall in love," because this overwhelmingly pleasurable state imbues even routine experiences with sparkly joy. In the beginning of a love affair, the pattern of brain activity recorded by an fMRI is virtually indistinguishable from that showing the effects of cocaine.[4] We eventually adapt to this state of bliss and find our feet back on the ground. As long as the stimulus (our lover) remains present, things feel just fine—a new normal. But if our lover wants a break or otherwise opts out of the relationship, an opponent process results in heartbreak. It can take months or years—depending on the intensity and duration of the partnership—to get back to a neutral feeling state.

Having a set point enables meaningful interpretation of a stream of ceaselessly changing input. Sustained feelings in either direction impede our ability to perceive and thus respond to new information, so the nervous system imposes transience. This means that if something truly wonderful happens—you meet Prince or Princess Charming—the elation will not last. On the other hand, even the most terrible calamity won't result in perpetual despair. This is also true with more mundane stimuli: we can probably all relate to the letdown after returning home from a great vacation, or to the flood of relief after a near accident on our commute.

It may seem curious, and certainly inconvenient, that rather than slowly letting a signal fade away, the brain counteracts it by producing its own in the opposite direction. To help appreciate the necessity of such an arrangement, let's imagine an alternate world where Tuesdays are designated "Happy Day" and all people have their feeling states artificially inflated on a weekly basis. While we would undoubtedly look forward to these days, events needing our attention would likely be missed or ignored on Tuesdays. Suppose that a child is injured, or a weather event becomes life threatening on Tuesday? Being blissed-out once a week could be a recipe for extinction. Persistently depressed states carry an analogous risk. We'd be unable to detect or act upon potential opportunities if we were in a state of chronic despair.

Information is detected, conveyed, and perceived by brain cells in terms of contrast from activity that is clamped at a "signature" (or characteristic) level, and can be either slowed down (inhibited) or sped up (excited) in response. The outcome for our feeling state is that it is stable over the long run—though not static. While different people may have different set points, for any individual the neutral state is robustly maintained throughout life. Happy-go-lucky kids tend to be contented adults, and pessimists generally remain so whatever their circumstances.

The fact that our feeling states are so tightly constrained has important implications for drug users, but before we get into those, it may be worth noting the few exceptions to this general tendency. Stroke victims with damage in specific cortical regions (especially in the right hemisphere) may turn from lifelong pessimists into optimists (or, with left hemisphere damage, the other way around). Other diseases, such as Alzheimer's, may produce similarly dramatic changes. Though for regular drug users affective stability makes it impossible to maintain a high, chronic use of stimulants like cocaine or methamphetamine may actually modify the affective set point. Unfortunately for users, this alteration is always in the "wrong" direction, resulting in lower baseline mood.

Homeostasis

So, we see that in addition to serving as a sensor, contrast detector, and coordinator of responses to environmental perturbations, the CNS is exquisitely capable of changing itself to adapt to environmental input. **In fact, the brain's capacities to dynamically respond to environmental stimuli and even to anticipate them (more on that later) are its most distinctive feature.**

Neurobiologists refer to the brain's capacity for modification as "plasticity," and it is the focus of intense research.* Persistent

---

* The term "plasticity" is used by neuroscientists to refer to the ability of the brain to modify its structure and function. Though changes are always possible (that is, we remain somewhat plastic until the day we die), they are

change in response to environmental input is called learning, and all organisms with a CNS—from cockroaches to the Dalai Lama—learn. As it turns out, memories, which are traces of learning, serve as Joe's escape from the terror and tedium of his helpless consciousness in a hospital bed in *Johnny Got His Gun*. They are also, in a manner of speaking, the neural cause of addiction.

The learning associated with addiction begins upon the very first exposure to a drug. So anyone who has ever tried a drug has experienced the brain's adaptive capacities. Adaptation begins immediately and, for example, causes a poor night's sleep after drinking as well as the feeling of general unease that characterizes a hangover the next day. These rebound states occur as brain cells, counteracting the activity-dampening effects of a few drinks, become more excited than normal. So, on the day after drinking, normal lighting seems too bright, and feelings of anxiety supplant feelings of relaxation. In this example, the effects of adaptation usually last less than twenty-four hours.

The term "tachyphylaxis" (TACKY-phil-axis), meaning "acute tolerance," refers to the adaptive, compensatory changes that begin as soon as alcohol reaches the brain. A large and rather arcane literature surrounding tachyphylaxis has a practical implication that, were it widely known, might be a real boon to DUI defense lawyers and their clients. It turns out that there is a reliable and interesting twist in the relationship between blood alcohol level and impairment, due to tachyphylaxis.

When someone drinks, alcohol levels in the blood increase as the drug is absorbed from the gut. Meanwhile, in the liver, alcohol is broken down (metabolized) at a steady rate. Thus, a bal-

---

especially likely during periods of rapid development, until the age of about twenty-five years.

ance of absorption into the blood and metabolism in the liver determines the concentration in the brain. If one were to graphically describe the changes in alcohol concentration over time during heavy drinking, the graph would look like an inverted U. No surprises here, but it turns out that the effects of alcohol are very much dependent on whether blood concentrations are increasing or falling. If we were to investigate impairment at two different times with *identical* alcohol concentrations in the same individual, one on the rising arm and the other on the falling arm of the curve, dramatic differences would be evident.

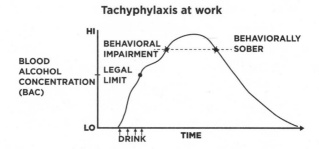

Tachyphylaxis at work

During the rising phase of the curve, the drinker experiences the pleasure resulting from mesolimbic activation. But at the same time, motor impairments such as stumbling gait and slowed speech grow increasingly pronounced. Later, when alcohol levels are falling, both pleasure and impairment are greatly reduced.

Researchers have spent quite a lot of time and effort studying these changes and have found that adaptations underlying tolerance occur with all drugs that affect the nervous system, and with similar rapidity. Virtually as soon as a drug begins to act on the brain, the brain begins to adapt—to counteract—that action. Thus, there is good rationale for arguing that despite a high BAC (blood alcohol concentration), because you are in a state of tachyphylaxis, you are really okay to drive. Good luck persuading the judge!

In this example, we see that tolerance accrues in a single session, even within a few minutes of exposure. Nicotine is another classic example of acute tolerance. The first cigarette of the day is the best one because after the particular brain sites for nicotine's effects have been activated, they become insensitive to subsequent exposures.

The brain learns by adapting to every drug that affects its function. Some of these changes are relatively transient, like tachyphylaxis in an occasional drinker, but as learning is stronger with repetition, chronic exposure to a drug results in more lasting alterations. For some drugs, such as antidepressants, adaptation is actually the therapeutic point. Developing tolerance to selective serotonin reuptake inhibitors (SSRIs) may help to change a pathological affective "set point" so that being depressed is no longer the patient's normal state. With abused drugs, however, such changes are a real drag. As the brain adapts to a drug of abuse and the drug becomes less effective at stimulating dopamine transmission, a user must take more and more to produce the same high. Engaged in a futile attempt to replicate the initial experiences, an addict repeatedly administering the drug ensures more and more adaptation. Cocaine addiction demonstrates this desperate state starkly: addicts feel compelled to use, often despite full knowledge of the tremendous social, economic, and personal costs. Abstinence, to the user's well-adapted mesolimbic circuitry, feels uninspired and hopeless, but a bump of cocaine doesn't produce as much of a high in this lower-than-normal baseline state. Eventually, the best the addict can hope for is transient alleviation of chronic despair.

A Working Model

Once while I was giving a brief lecture on Solomon and Corbit's opponent-process theory to a group of high school students, a young man abruptly leaped to his feet and exclaimed, "This changes my life!" I share his sentiments and wish all teaching were so rewarding. But this theory is also scientifically important because it has largely set the course for the way scientists think about and study addiction.

The essence of the theory is depicted in the following figures. Solomon and Corbit use the terms "State A" and "State B" to refer to opposing affective experiences. The feelings produced by a stimulus are captured in State A, and the rebound caused by the attempted return to the neutral state is depicted in State B. Depending on the initial stimulus, State A can be either pleasant or unpleasant, but whatever it is, State B is the opposite. At first, there is a large change, which is tempered by adaptation but stays in the A-zone until the stimulus is turned off, at which point we experience the opposite state (think of the response to alcohol). Our net experience, shown in the solid line, involves two entirely different neural processes. The *a process* is the neural response to the stimulus. If we are talking about drug use, we can think of the *a process* as what the drug does to the brain. Big doses produce large *a processes,* and protracted stimuli produce long-lasting *a processes.* But for each *a process,* there is a *b process.* The *b process* is the brain's response to the *a process,* or the brain's response to what the drug does to the brain, counteracting the changes in neural activity produced by the stimulus in an effort to return brain activity to its neutral, homeostatic state.

When the brain is first exposed to a stimulus, the *a process* is unmitigated by compensatory brain mechanisms, and

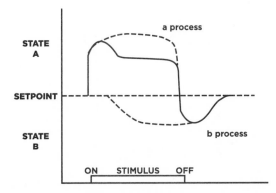

Our experience (solid line) is the combined effect of the drug (*a process*) and the brain's opponent response to the drug (*b process*).

thus State A is experienced in full. However, as the *b process* is recruited, State A is dampened. This arrangement leads to an initial peak experience followed by a leveling off. While the *a process* is a direct reflection of the stimulus and so is always the same if the stimulus is the same (a certain number of ounces of alcohol or milligrams of heroin, for instance), this is not so with the compensatory *b process*. Generated by a powerfully adaptive nervous system, the *b process* learns with time and exposure. Repeated encounters with the stimulus result in faster, bigger, and longer-lasting *b processes* that are better able to maintain homeostasis in the face of disruption. Moreover, the *b process* can be elicited solely by environmental stimuli that promise the *a process* is coming—which is what happened with Pavlov's dogs, who learned to salivate even when food was not present.

I don't have any tattoos, but on my short list, if I decide to get one, is a figure like the one shown below, also copied from Solomon and Corbit's seminal paper and illustrating the changes that occur in the *b process* as a result of adaptation. Note how the experience of the stimulus is dramatically altered, so that

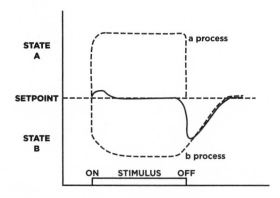

As a result of adaptation after repeated drug taking, the opponent process becomes quicker, stronger, and longer lasting—leading to a reduction in the subjective experience (tolerance) and withdrawal and craving when the drug is not present.

now there is hardly a bump in feeling state. In many ways, this figure is the theoretical heart of scientific understanding about addiction and the core of this book, depicting how the drug comes to function mainly to stave off withdrawal and craving in the face of the brain's powerful ability to counteract perturbation. It also explains why the states of withdrawal and craving from any drug are *always* exactly opposite to the drug's effects. If a drug makes you feel relaxed, withdrawal and craving are experienced as anxiety and tension. If a drug helps you wake up, adaptation includes lethargy; if it reduces pain sensations, suffering will be your lot.

My clever undergraduates are quick to point out a flip side to Solomon and Corbit's model: if you want to achieve a sustained positive state, you could submit yourself to negatively charged experiences. This way the opponent process would be positive. Solomon and Corbit argued that such a pattern may be at work in an activity like skydiving. Jumping out of an airplane at several thousand feet produces intense feelings of arousal and panic, even feelings associated with impending death. They would probably last for much of the air time and certainly for all of the "free fall." As the stimulus ends and your feet are miraculously back on solid ground, not only is the panic gone, but according to hobbyists it is like being awash in feelings of extreme calm and well-being. The relief following an intensely stressful experience, if you live through the event, may make it all worthwhile. Maybe this helps explain why people push themselves to exercise or go to graduate school.

The hallmarks of addiction—tolerance, withdrawal, and craving—are captured in the consequences of the *b process*. Tolerance occurs because more drug is needed to produce an *a process* capable of overcoming a stronger and stronger *b process*. Withdrawal happens because the *b process* outlasts the drug's effects. And craving is virtually guaranteed because any environmental signal that has been associated with the drug can itself elicit a *b process* that can only be assuaged by indulging in the drug. This might happen at cocktail hour, during stressful times, or even upon awakening if that's when you typically start using; in particular contexts such as bars or family gatherings; or in the presence of specific cues such as spoons, dealers, and paychecks, which is one of the reasons intense feelings of craving continue to frustrate recovery. To this day, and seemingly out of the blue, a certain warmth and humidity in the air or a specific type of music can make my mouth pucker with the anticipation of tequila.

In other words, the brain is so well organized to counteract perturbations that it uses its exceptional learning skills to anticipate disruptions, rather than wait for the changes themselves, and begins to dampen drug effects before the drug has even been delivered. Suppose you enjoy a few drinks with friends at a neighborhood bar every Friday after work, as you have been doing for years. It turns out that the predictability of this routine leads to changes in your experience. First, the alcohol will have less effect on you in that particular place and time and with those particular friends than it would have elsewhere. If you changed plans and went instead to a party, you'd become more intoxicated with the same amount to drink.

This tendency for environmental cues to induce craving has been recognized for a long time. In the mid-nineteenth century, Robert Macnish, a Scottish surgeon, commented, in his book *The Anatomy of Drunkenness,*[5] on the learning he observed in some of his alcoholic patients:

> Man is very much the creature of habit. By drinking regularly at certain times he feels the longing for liquor at the stated return of these periods—as after dinner, or immediately before going to bed, or whatever period that may be. He even finds it in certain companies, or in a particular tavern at which he is in the habit of taking his libations.

So, returning to the present-day bar scene: let's imagine that you're taking antibiotics and you plan not to drink that night. Having had a good day, you're upbeat as you walk into the pub, anticipating a nice evening unwinding with friends. Chances are that your fine mood will dissipate and tension and irritability will mount. The sights, sounds, and smells of the bar have elicited the *b process,* and your sober evening is likely to include feelings of craving and withdrawal.

Treatment programs now take heed of cue-induced relapse. In the 1970s, therapeutic communities were a popular treatment strategy. Addicts would be transplanted to a totally different context—say a goat farm in the country—far away from their urban home to spend several months or even years practicing a sober life. By the time they'd leave the community, they'd feel free from the pernicious craving to use. As a result, they and their counselors and family members would be full of optimism as they resumed their former lives. And things would usually go well for some time, until a chance meeting with an old using buddy, passage by a favorite bar, or the sight of a hypodermic needle in a doctor's office would elicit a *b process,* precipitating an "inexplicable" relapse.

Cutting-edge treatments take almost the opposite tact from the pastoral setting strategy (unless of course your using primarily took place on the farm). Following detox and some stability in mood and physiology (usually after several weeks of clean time), the addict is purposely exposed to cues that used to coincide with using, but this time within a supportive, therapeutic context. Wads of cash, drawing fluid into a syringe, or experiencing a disappointing day at first is likely to produce profound physiological and psychological effects such as changes in heart rate, body temperature, and mood. But with repeated exposure (and no drug delivery), such responses indicative of the *b process* begin to dissipate and eventually disappear. So, it is possible to extinguish a craving over time, as the brain adapts again, but this time to the non-predictive value of the cues.

Addiction Is a Consequence of Normal Brain Functioning

Addiction differs in many ways from diseases typical of the broad category, a fact that took me several years to appreciate. Though I believed—and still do—that it is a brain disorder, it's not like having a tumor or Alzheimer's disease. Both of these can be definitively diagnosed by identifying particular cellular changes. Diabetes or high cholesterol is even easier to assess—by a simple blood test—and obesity is determined by a body mass index. On the other hand, there are no clear-cut tests to determine whether one is, or is not, an addict, and in addition to making diagnosis murky, this lack of clarity hinders efforts to cure the disease. If we remove the tumor or other errant structures, restore an appropriate insulin response, or lose enough weight, related diseases might indeed be cured. In the case of addiction—really a disorder of thought, emotion, and behavior resulting from widespread adaptation in multiple brain circuits—a cure is unlikely aside from removing most of the matter above my shoulders. The tenacity of addiction is as evident to researchers and clinicians as it is to addicts. I've been clean for more than thirty years, and I'm still not really interested in moderation. Often people ask whether I don't wish I might have a glass of wine or a hit off a joint, but I don't want just one glass or a light buzz; I want the whole bottle, the bag, and then some more of each. The Grateful Dead argued that "too much of everything is just enough," but as it turned out for Jerry Garcia, and I'd bet is the case for many of us, too much is still not enough. In other words, if by chance someone does develop a pill to cure my addictive nature, I'd take two and use every day.

There are many contributors to this tendency toward excess, but ultimately my behavior is extreme because the stimuli (that is, drugs) have had such a potent impact on me relative to natural stimuli. The nervous system of an addict is acting normally and predictably in response to such consequential input, and addiction is a natural consequence. It's also not likely to be prevented by anything less than preventing learning and memory. However, this would defeat the purpose because you could only get high if you weren't aware of it.

The irony here will not be lost on most of us. Addicts don't use on a regular basis because they are addicted; they are addicted because they use a lot, and regularly. The lackadaisical habits of so-called normal people who leave drinks half finished, snort a few lines on a Friday night, or occasionally smoke a cigarette with friends are strikingly different from those of addicts. Though adaptation still occurs in "chippers," it is virtually imperceptible because of the irregular and low-dose patterns of use.

I was clean for close to two years and had been volunteering in my biopsychology professor's laboratory to get some research experience. One part of the protocol required daily administration of an experimental drug into the subjects' (rats') peritoneum, which is the sac that loosely constrains the abdominal organs. The standard procedure is to cup the rat gently in one hand, insert the needle with the other, and create negative pressure by pulling slightly back on the needle to be sure the injection isn't going straight into a blood vessel. I thought I'd fully extinguished any personal associations with needles, having performed hundreds of injections by this time, but one day when I pulled back and the needle filled with blood, I heard clamorous ringing in my ears and a taste in my mouth that were characteristic of cocaine going into *my* vein. It was years later, in a completely different context, and I had not a whit of desire to use at that moment, but just seeing blood filling the syringe caused an instantaneous reaction. I let my colleague finish the injections and went back to my dorm sobered by the astounding power of memory.

3

One Salient Example: THC

If all the year were playing holidays,
To sport would be as tedious as to work,
But when they seldom come, they wished
*   for come,*
And nothing pleaseth but rare accidents.

—William Shakespeare, *Henry IV, Part 1*

Drug of Choice

From the moment I drank the wine in my friend's basement
until I got clean and sober, I didn't turn down a single opportunity to use any drug. People often ask about a "drug of choice."
To me this is an ambiguous concept. I, and hordes of people like
me, will use virtually anything, depending on circumstances.
In truth I'd choose them all, sometimes serially and sometimes
all at once; I wasn't picky. A few of my choices were toxic, others stupid or pointless, and some absolutely terrific. However,
if the question were stated this way: "You're going to a desert
island to live out the rest of your life and can only take one substance, what would it be?" Without hesitation, I'd choose a limitless supply of weed (and some seeds just in case). A friend once
commented that I chain-smoked the drug, and she was right.
From the first delicious bong hits of the day until the final joint,

I loved the taste, the smell, and the fabulous buffering effects separating me from the messy business of interacting with other people and fulfilling my daily obligations as, at the same time, weed lent promise of something new and glittering in the midst of the unappealing present. As an antidote to boredom, the drug made everything more interesting, and time and space delightful instead of threatening. An introvert to begin with, I loved spending hours stoned on the beach searching for shells and listening to lapping waves, a thoroughly engrossing way to pass the time.

Not to belabor the point, but in many ways my relationship with the drug was among the purest and most wonderful relationships of my life. From the first time I got high until long after I'd smoked my last bowl, I loved marijuana like a best friend. This is not hyperbole. Some people it makes sleepy, others paranoid (due, no doubt, to an unfortunate confluence of neurobiology and genetics), but for me it was nearly perfect. One of my favorite moments was shortly after coming to consciousness in a new day and seeing for an instant the vast bleakness of life before me and then suddenly realizing—just as newlyweds might reach in excitement and hope for a spouse beside them in bed—that I could get high. The first few hits of the day were reliably comforting as the gray dust of reality was blown away to reveal beauty and meaning in everyday encounters. My lover and I were in on a secret, and as far as I was concerned, there was nothing that would ever come between us.

This I mean literally, and I have dozens of examples of stupid or risky or selfish behavior that I engaged in to maintain my supply. One time during a rare dry spell, I decided to address my rising sense of anxiety with a trip to Nickeltown (so named because for $5 you could pick up a small envelope with enough weed for a joint or two). To me this was like tourist shopping at a high-priced market; I knew I would be ripped off, but I was coming out of my skin and anything was better than nothing. Greedily arriving at my apartment, I ripped open the bag to find *pine needles.* I was furious, ranting and raving, waking my roommates (who had chosen to simply drink themselves to sleep), until I finally decided I'd drive back to 'town and straighten things out! I might have been only nineteen or twenty and lacking in both offensive and defensive resources, but I was full of indignation and desperation, so back I went. I arrived after midnight, and the streets were deserted (because there was nothing to sell, I now suspect, but I wasn't able to make this connection at the time and could only surmise that someone was holding out). Anyway, I parked in an intersection, turned on my brights, and laid on the horn. People began yelling from their windows, but I yelled right back: "GIVE ME MY POT!" This continued for a bit, until rocks and bottles began denting my car. I finally left, seething and sobbing, full of self-righteous anger, unable to see beyond my own need. I learned from this experience to be sure to keep a hidden stash for such emergencies.

Why So Special?

If alcohol is a pharmacological sledgehammer and cocaine a laser (and they are), marijuana is a bucket of red paint. This is so for at least two reasons. First is its well-known ability to accentuate attributes of environmental stimuli: music is amazing, food delicious, jokes hilarious, colors rich, and so on. Second, its effects are neither precise nor specific, but modulatory and widespread. It's a five-gallon bucket with a four-inch brush, painting up the gain on all kinds of neural processing. Unlike cocaine, for instance, which acts in relatively few discrete spots in the brain, THC (or delta-9-tetrahydrocannabinol), the active ingredient in marijuana, acts throughout the brain, and in some regions in every single connection (of which there are trillions). The broad reach of this drug was a big surprise to researchers when it was realized in the early 1990s. I was in graduate school at the time, and the news was so momentous that—in the way that some people remember where they were and what they were doing when Kennedy was shot or the Twin Towers came down—I remember my exact circumstances when the receptor for THC was cloned. A receptor is the bit of protein found on the surface of cells that, when activated by a drug or neurotransmitter, confers its effects. The drug without the receptor protein would be completely inert, but interactions of THC with its receptor, at least in my case, made existence bearable.

The first time I smoked pot might have been the most unadulterated fun in my entire life. I laughed until my face and my sides ached; everything was absolutely hilarious yet worthy of deep thought—what could be better? A friend had gotten a joint from her older brother, and we smoked it by an abandoned house on our way to the mall. I didn't feel anything at first, but about twenty minutes later, exactly coincident with walking into the shopping center, we were both simultaneously overcome, and high indeed! I now know that the delay happens because of sponge-like binding proteins that are floating around in the blood, to which THC molecules are attracted like magnets; they can't affect the brain until these proteins are fully saturated. Once all the binding sites are occupied, though, THC can finally be distributed to the brain. I've heard that some people don't get any effects from the drug, and though this is theoretically possible, it's extremely unlikely. More likely they need to smoke a little more.

Of course, we didn't evolve the machinery to produce these complicated receptor proteins or spend the energy to put them all over the brain just in case someone offers us a hit. So the seeming allover effects of THC led researchers on a hunt for the endogenous transmitter that THC must be mimicking. But searching for a transmitter is like looking for an acquaintance when you're not sure which neighborhood, city, or state the person lives in. Receptors, like houses, are easier to find because they are larger and less likely to be moving around.

So first we had to locate the receptor, and to do that, researchers tagged THC molecules with a radioactive label and injected them into a rat. After time enough for the drug to distribute, the animal was humanely sacrificed, and very thin slices of brain tissue were mounted to slides and rinsed thoroughly so that only the THC that was associated with a receptor remained; all the unbound or free drug was removed. Much to everyone's surprise, the THC was interacting with receptors all over the brain—on the cortex, the structure involved in information processing and other kinds of thinking and awareness, but also in many deeper subcortical structures having to do with emotion and motivation. There were differences in the density of the receptors, with some areas expressing fewer interaction sites, but others were virtually opaque with binding.[1]

This was perhaps the first finding (of many to follow) demonstrating the unique characteristics of the endocannabinoid system (endocannabinoid stands for endogenous cannabis). If we did the same experiment with radioactively labeled cocaine, we'd find far fewer places where the drug stuck, and they'd be more sparsely distributed. Even the opioid system, which is incredibly rich and complex (and utilized by all narcotics like

CB₁ receptors

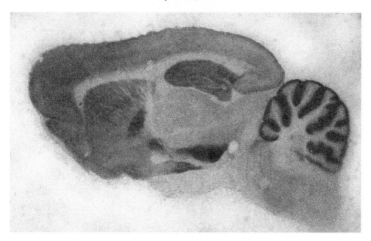

THC acts throughout the brain in trillions of synapses by interacting with CB₁ receptors labeled darkly.

heroin, OxyContin, and morphine), is nowhere near as densely and widely distributed as the endocannabinoid pathways.

My labmates and I thought that there had been some mistake with the assay. How could the receptors for this drug be all over the surface of the brain as well as in virtually every subcortical structure? More important, what was the natural THC-like compound, and what was its function?

Research is still ongoing and continues to be exciting because the field is relatively new, but we do know that the initial binding studies were correct: THC modulates activity in a huge number of synapses, in almost every brain structure. Its primary receptor in the brain is called CB_1 for cannabinoid receptor 1. The wide and dense distribution of CB_1 receptors has profound implications. Instead of producing specific effects—as dopamine does, for instance, in signaling news and stimulating movement—whatever activates CB_1 was likely to have general effects, by influencing neurotransmission all over the brain. But before we could prove it, we had to learn more about the overall cannabinoid system.

The first natural chemical found in the brain to activate the receptor was termed anandamide, which is a Sanskrit word conveying "bliss." The other primary endocannabinoid is 2-AG (or 2-arachidonoylglycerol). Cannabinoid transmitters and their transmission in the brain are atypical. For one thing, classic neurotransmitters are stored in vesicles (membranous sacs) and released from the terminal ends of nerve cells (neurons), where they diffuse across a little gap called a synapse and interact with receptors on an adjacent cell. In contrast, anandamide and 2-AG communicate in the opposite direction, diffusing "upstream" across the synapse to convey information from the receiving to the sending cell. Once they reach their target, CB_1 receptors on the first cell's surface, they produce their actions, which essentially are to alter the signal-to-noise relationship so that the message conveyed by classical neurotransmitters in this synapse carries more import.

The influence of the endocannabinoids is still being carefully investigated, and the details are complex to say the least, but my view of the literature is that anandamide and 2-AG act as a sort of exclamation point on neural communication, indicating that whatever the message just transmitted across the synapse, it was important.

What does all this intracellular back-and-forth have to do with our experience? In the mid-1970s, especially in suburban settings like mine, malls were about the only place to find autonomy if you were a kid. My friend and I had been there many times, so I'm sure our overwhelming experience of delight and joy had nothing to do with the wholly predictable environment. However, it sure seemed so! The sounds and sights were so incredibly stimulating: mundane department stores were transformed into rich playgrounds, and the smells in the food court were amazing. At one point, suddenly ravenous, we hit the pizza parlor, and to say this was the best slice of pizza of my life is an understatement. It was profoundly delicious! Everything was so much better than normal.

It seems that anandamide and similar compounds evolved along with the CB_1 receptor to modulate normal activity, highlighting important neurotransmission. The normal activity of the brain, as we've discussed, mediates all of our experiences, thoughts, behaviors, and emotions. The cannabinoid system helps to sort our experiences, indicating which are the most meaningful or salient. The system activates naturally to distinguish input that might contribute to our flourishing—for instance, a good source of food, a potential mate, or other meaningful connections, information, or stimuli. Anandamide and 2-AG and their receptor are all over the brain because such input might be carried in any number of pathways, depending on the exact nature of the stimulus. For example, let's say one day you are exploring your surroundings somewhat aimlessly, when you serendipitously begin following a route that eventually leads to something good. The millions of neurons involved in this discovery—including those involved in processing input from your senses, stimulating movement, coding memories or thoughts connecting this good thing to your plans or communicating it to others—are likely all releasing cannabinoids to turn up the volume on this information, helping to distinguish it from the other parts of your day in which interactions with the environment weren't all that special.

This should make it easy to understand why the stimuli we encounter when stoned are so intensely rich. Sights, sounds, tastes, and thoughts that might otherwise be average take on incredible attributes. Early in my love affair with pot, I remember finding Rice-A-Roni so astoundingly delicious I couldn't imagine how it stayed on the shelves of the grocery stores. Today

I'd have to be backpacking for at least a week before I'd even find it palatable, but with my synapses primed for import, food is exceptional, music transcendent, concepts mind-blowing. What a wonderful treat this is, especially for someone who dreads the humdrum!

Unfortunately, there is a dark side to all this neural spotlighting. If everything is highlighted as meaningful, then nothing can really stand out. What use is a watering can after all, if the fields are flooded? The lack of contrast disables the sorting machinery that helps us make sense of our environment by separating relevant from irrelevant. After one comes down, the lack of sorting makes it hard to recall the wonderful urgency of those experiences.

The other downside is that on rare occasions when I was not high, I could barely feign interest in anything. The world on the drug seemed so much shinier than the world without it. One bright sunny day I was driving south on I-95, somehow lost my grip, and the joint I was smoking went flying out of the car. It was most of a nice fat spliff, and I didn't think twice before pulling off the road and walking the shoulder against six lanes of speeding traffic. It seems a little crazy to me now, but at the time I was determined. When I lost my grandmother's engagement ring, I took it less seriously. Of course, I found the roach.

Consequences

After I got sober, it took me a little over a year to go a single day without wishing for a drink, but it was more than *nine years* before my craving to get high abated. For the longest time, I couldn't go to indoor concerts, especially if I was in proximity to pot. Good sinsemilla would induce a sort of mini panic attack. I'd get sweaty and anxious and have to leave. During this nearly decade-long purgatory, I broke up with a pretty good guy (great cook, decent skier) only because he occasionally wanted to get high. Though it was not even around me, I was unable to bear the idea that he'd be somewhere laughing his ass off, while I'd be missing out. It sounds ridiculous now, but I hope it's perfectly clear that while I like all drugs, pot I adore.

Predictably, chronic exposure leads to substantial consequences. The brain adapts by downregulating the cannabinoid system.[2] "Downregulation" is a general term describing processes that work to ensure homeostasis, which in this case translates to a dramatic reduction in the number and sensitivity of CB_1 receptors. Without copious amounts of pot on board, everything is dull and uninspiring.

Downregulation of CB_1

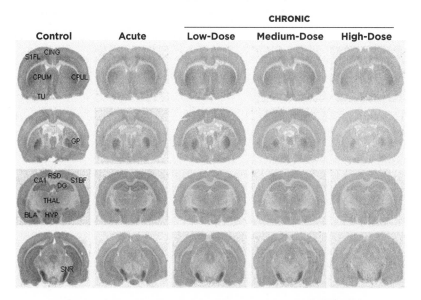

The left column shows slices from the brain of a rat treated with a placebo. Dark spots indicate CB_1 receptors. A single (acute) exposure to a THC analog causes downregulation of receptors. The three columns of chronic exposure show dose-dependent downregulation after fourteen days of treatment.

There's been a long-standing debate, akin to one about the relationship between cancer and smoking in many ways, about whether regular marijuana smoking leads to an amotivational syndrome ("amotivational" means lacking motivation). For instance, does regular use lead to spending long hours on the couch watching cartoons, or does it just so happen that people who like to sit around watching television (or poring through shells at the beach) also enjoy marijuana? Because correlation doesn't mean causation, cigarette companies argued for decades that a predisposition for cancer and the tendency to inhale cigarette smoke just coincidentally occur in the same people. In both cases, common sense and mounting evidence point to the same thing. Downregulation of CB_1 receptors might make the user more suitable for jobs that don't require creativity or innovation, exactly the effects that initial exposure seemed to stimulate.

My first few months without pot were especially miserable. Though I was in a new environment, with new friends and countless novel experiences, I remember very little and experienced everything as bland beyond belief (in addition to feeling anxious, depressed, and ashamed). However, about three months into my new drug-free life, I was walking along a street in Minneapolis and nearly fell to my knees, struck by the brilliance of the fall foliage. All around me were a million bright oranges, reds, yellows, and greens; I must have felt the way the first viewers of movies in Technicolor did. Where had all this come from? In fact, downregulation had reversed with my abstinence. As my receptors returned, so did my appreciation for everyday beauty.

Fortunately, after nine long years pining away, I realized one day that I didn't crave marijuana. For the next twenty years or so, I relished my freedom! I could be around weed without feeling like the last one sitting at a dance. And then I entered perimenopause and really understood why the drug was on the planet. Though I hadn't smoked in thirty years, I just knew it would be a perfect antidote to the irritability, hypersensitivity, and frustration with daily tasks that accompanied my transition. During the first few years of plummeting hormones, not only would I have given my left arm to smoke; I'd have cut it off myself and felt as if I'd gotten a decent deal. The craving not only came back but had somehow matured. I even fantasized I would get cancer and a doctor would deem the prescription necessary. Hmmm, a life-threatening illness, but I could toke away! The reason I didn't start smoking despite my desire was that I knew the delicious escape it would afford me would come at a cost. The things about my life that I'd come to enjoy—my intellectual work, family, and other ambitions and hobbies—would grow pale in comparison to sitting around smoking a bowl.

I have a friend and colleague, a smart professor at a good university, who used to like to drink a lot but was finding some of the effects embarrassing if not disabling. He switched to smoking pot. He and his wife put the kids to bed and relax together by getting high. He started to notice that if he smoked a little before doing his "daddy duties" he was, as he described it, a more engaged parent. With just a couple of hits, he was able to play more with his children and didn't find the carpool, meal preparation, or team coaching quite so irritating and tedious. "Great," I said. "How's it with your kids when you're not high?" "Increasingly irritating and tedious," he admitted.

So, if you smoke weed, remember that infrequent and intermittent use is the best way to prevent downregulation and its unfortunate effects: tolerance, dependence, and a loss of interest in the unenhanced world.

4

Dream Weavers: Opiates

> If you think dope is for kicks and for
> thrills, you're out of your mind. There
> are more kicks to be had in a good case
> of paralytic polio or by living in an iron
> lung. If you think you need stuff to play
> music or sing, you're crazy. It can fix
> you so you can't play nothing or sing
> nothing.
>
> —Billie Holiday (1915–1959)

A Love Story

The tale of opiate users is one of such great love and such great suffering as to make *Romeo and Juliet* seem like a middle school melodrama. This class of drugs delivers heartbreak like no other, initially providing a sense of security and well-being that soon transmutes into something like being stranded on a barren moonscape without oxygen.

In the beginning, opiates are an ideal other. As they beckon graciously, it feels entirely natural to respond with trust and gratitude. Unlike stimulants, or even alcohol, the subjective effects of these drugs seem almost perfectly subtle as they bestow utter contentment. At first the relationship is fun and easy, polishing up cloudy afternoons that might otherwise be irksome and muting broken edges of disappointment. As with requited love, the myopic sense of contentment in opiate's embrace is like an island vacation or a trip along a golden road; everything superfluous to the relationship recedes to a distant horizon. So what that life is full of small hurts and insults, because the perfect antidote can be readily found in a pill or bag. If only it could stay this way!

But, alas, for reasons that seem cruelly capricious, the drug becomes fickle just as your longing grows increasingly urgent. "Darling!" you whisper and then cry, "Please? *Please, please!*" What has happened? Why can't you experience the perfect solace you once shared? Smack is all you care about as the intimacy you shared gives way to hopeful longing and then to deep grief and finally to bleak isolation. Because your lover had been so perfectly attentive, the devastation is immense, and your heartbreak inconsolable. Desperate and foolish, you'll degrade yourself however you must to experience even a shred of what you once had.

But there will be no happy reunion as your lover remains distant, if not oblivious, to your agony. The rare meet ups are unsatisfying, hampered by a sure knowledge that they won't last. So you suffer for days, weeks, months, and even years, tortured by the somatic and psychic memories of merciful encounters along with the sure knowledge that you've been expelled from the garden. Wandering through the wreckage of your former life, you can't seem to recall anything of value. You suffer, in proportion to the duration and intensity of your relationship, as you seek a way of returning to the first precious moments of falling in love.

Trending Appetites

Narcotics—the umbrella term for all opiate drugs—are very much on our collective mind these days, if not in our blood, as the tragedy of opiate addiction is enacted thousands of times a day, all over the world.

More than one in five Americans takes opiates during their lifetime, either illegally or by prescription, or both, and as the second most addictive drug (behind nicotine) the consequences of opiate abuse are impossible not to notice. A surge in the number of lethal opiate-related deaths as well as several recent high-profile cases (Prince, Heath Ledger, and Philip Seymour Hoffman, for example) have helped call attention to the problem, though the phenomenon is not new. Janis Joplin, John Belushi, Sid Vicious, Jim Morrison, Judy Garland, and even Elvis Presley also died as a result of opiate abuse. The use of these drugs has been on the rise over the past few years, however, and more people now die of narcotic overdoses than automobile accidents.

Many of these people begin their addiction in a doctor's office. In 2012, 259 million prescriptions were written for opioids, which was more than enough to give every American adult his or her own bottle of pills. Naturally, such liberal prescribing is associated with a rise in lethal overdoses. Among women, who are most likely to take these medications (partly because they are more likely to suffer from chronic pain), the first decade of the twenty-first century saw a 400 percent increase in lethal overdoses. And even those who live through a near-death experience are unlikely to stop using. A recent study found that 91 percent who overdose on medication continue to refill their prescriptions. As the cold blue bodies pile up, governments, local law enforcement, and family members wring their hands in dismay.

Who's to blame for this situation? The truth is, we all contribute to the prevalence of these drugs in our communities by swallowing whole the illusion that suffering is avoidable by some outside "fix." Together with our doctors, we've been in collective denial about the fact that these drugs are unable to provide a sustainable solution to the pains of living, and therefore the only real beneficiaries are the pushers, in this case, the pharmaceutical companies.

Heroin and other street opiates show parallel trends, with about a 40 percent increase in use *each year* since 2010. The vast majority of new heroin users (about four out of five) start by misusing prescription painkillers and turn to street narcotics because they are cheaper and easier to get. Unfortunately, there's no regulation of illicit substances (by definition), and the purity varies tremendously. As a consequence, the rate of overdose deaths from street narcotics nearly quadrupled from 2000 to 2013 and by all accounts is continuing to rise.

If we widen our lens, big swings in the popularity of all illicit drugs are readily evident. For instance, narcotics were also very popular in the United States during the mid-nineteenth century, particularly among Asian immigrants, women, and (believe it or not) children. During the ensuing years, there have been a number of surges in opiate use, generally within specific subpopulations—hipsters in the 1940s, beatniks in the 1950s, and Vietnam soldiers in the late 1960s and the 1970s. Overall use of opiates diminished in the 1980s and 1990s, because stimulants were a better fit with cultural values of productivity and efficiency, but today they are definitely back and embraced by adolescents and young adults in increasing proportions. So, it ought to be obvious that changing laws, medical practice, or the availability of an antidote (that is, antagonists like naltrexone or naloxone) won't win any drug wars. The drive to change our subjective experience is universal, and there are many like me who will try anything that might get us high. Therefore, the solution is not to be found on the supply side, but rather depends on a change in demand, and that's likely to be an inside job.

I tried opiates only a handful of times during my using career because with few exceptions they were not readily available in my time and place. I liked the experience, which, at the low to moderate doses I enjoyed, conveyed a sense of warmth and contentment. I'm fairly certain that the story would have been different if I'd been afforded the opportunity to inject these drugs.

It's hard to overestimate the power of the hold opiates come to have on their users. Several years ago, for example, I was conducting a study to assess the benefit of acupuncture treatment for heroin addicts at a detox in Portland, Oregon. The idea was that needling at "active sites" would release endorphins and thus ease the pain and suffering of withdrawal. Detoxing addicts who volunteered for the study were randomly assigned to either an active group or a placebo group (for whom needling occurred at spots purportedly lacking therapeutic benefit). Licensed acupuncturists delivered treatment each morning for about thirty minutes to all inpatients who volunteered for the study, and things seemed to be going well during the first few days of the experiment. Patients were asked to record their withdrawal symptoms several times a day using paper-and-pencil questionnaires, and there was a suggestion that those receiving active treatments were a little less anxious and slept better than did the placebo controls.

However, the study was unexpectedly cut short after a young addict who was known to most of the community checked out and promptly died with a needle in his arm. It took only a few hours after the news broke for the center to empty out entirely— not to mourn, but to score. The patients recognized in their friend's death a sign of high-quality dope. You've probably seen similar phenomena in your community; regional bursts in overdoses tend to occur not because most addicts don't know what's to be found but because they do. They are victims of the laws of pharmacology who fail to recognize that even drugs like fentanyl and carfentanil, which are thousands of times as potent as heroin, can't deliver the desired effects to a learned brain (though, unfortunately, they remain potent enough at depressing respiration, which is how they can be lethal).

Dream Makers

Addictive drugs are separated into different groups based primarily on their effects. Stimulants increase activity, hallucinogens alter perception, and sedative-hypnotics slow brain activity and promote sleep. Opiates or narcotics get their classification from a shared molecular structure and common effects, one of the most reliable of which is analgesia, or pain relief. Opiate compounds, initially derived from poppy plants, have been used for at least seven thousand years—beginning in Neolithic times—for both medicinal and recreational purposes (categories that are not always clearly delineated). These compounds are still the drug of choice for intense acute or chronic pain. But, as always, there are side effects. Some of these are respiratory depression (responsible for death by overdose), constipation (making it a useful treatment for severe diarrhea), and euphoria (an antidote, we might say, to dysphoria, another seemingly unavoidable aspect of the human condition). And, of course, it's this latter effect that gives the drug its addictive liability.

From a neuroscience perspective, the appeal of opiate drugs is easy to understand. The large class of narcotics, from heroin, fentanyl, and oxycodone to their less potent analogs like tramadol and codeine, all work by mimicking endorphins (*endoge-nous* m*orphine*-like substances), the body's natural painkillers. It turns out that our brains manufacture an incredibly rich and varied pharmacopoeia of these natural opioids, the sheer number and wide distribution of which suggest that they play a critical role in our survival.

A firsthand description suggests what that role might be. The explorer and missionary David Livingstone was on a trip to Africa when he was attacked by a lion. (He is familiar to many by the understated greeting he received from Henry Morton Stanley when Stanley finally located the missing Scot: "Dr. Livingstone, I presume?") Livingstone survived the mauling, and his account dramatically illustrates the role of endorphins in the body. The lion, he wrote, "caught me by the shoulder as he sprang, and we both came to the ground together. Growling horribly close to my ear, it shook me as a terrier dog does a rat. The shock . . . caused a dreaminess, in which there was no sense of pain nor feeling of terror, though quite conscious of all that was happening."[1]

We now know that his experience is fairly common (not the lion attack, obviously, but the relaxed dreamy state induced by stress or danger). Imagine, if you will, a present-day version of the lion attack experienced by Dr. Livingstone. Let's say that you are returning to your apartment after a long day at the office, only to be surprised by a masked intruder. In the scuffle, you suffer a deep gash from the intruder's knife. What to do?

Suppose you are overcome with pain and fear and spend what remains of your life writhing on the floor of your apartment until you bleed to death or are dispatched some other way. This is unlikely to help you survive or—more to the point— reproduce in the future. Instead, within about ninety seconds of the alarming encounter, cells in your brain will stimulate gene activity to direct the synthesis of endorphins, which are quickly released to produce effects throughout the central nervous system: blocking pain transmission, inhibiting the panic response, and hopefully facilitating an escape. It is easy to see how modulating pain and suffering would provide evolutionary advantage to an organism.

Another clue that natural opioids play important roles in survival is that the neurochemical family is so large and diverse. That indicates a long evolutionary history. There are dozens of different opioids manufactured by the brain (including actual morphine). Experiments have shown that these chemicals serve a range of critical functions including modulating activities like sex, attachment, and learning. It seems rather unlikely that Dr. Livingstone's Creator, however benevolent, would make such a rich palette of options just to help you die!

Yin and Yang

Most people are acquainted with endorphins, perhaps recognizing that these chemicals contribute to a "runner's high," the warm, sated feeling after eating spicy food, or sex-induced euphoria. But few people recognize that there is another, equally large family of natural compounds that evolved to *counteract* the endorphins. These have been collectively called anti-opiates, and they produce exactly the opposite effects as narcotics. Why did evolution or that benevolent Creator decide we need compounds that enhance suffering and restlessness?

Recall your virtual home invasion. Suppose you manage to escape from the intruder and get out onto the street, benefiting from a lovely flood of endorphins, despite your potentially life-threatening injury. Once you are no longer in immediate danger, it would actually be helpful to perceive your pain rather than to remain analgesic. Otherwise you might still die—just more slowly—from loss of blood or, eventually, infection. So the brain doesn't wait for the endorphins to naturally degrade. Instead, the edges of perception are sharpened by a flood of anti-opiates.

In fact, pain has two primary purposes: the first is to teach us to avoid dangerous stimuli or situations, and the second is to encourage recuperation after failing the first lesson. Another potential rationale for the existence of anti-opiates was outlined in earlier chapters: the brain's role as contrast detector relies upon a stable baseline. Anti-opiates restore the brain to its baseline most efficiently.

One of my colleagues, Eric Wiertelak, is among many scientists helping to shed light on the homeostatic system of opiates and their antis.[2] In a clever set of experiments, he trained rats to expect a stressful stimulus and after repeated trials found that the rats began to synthesize their own analgesics to help cope. He was able to identify the analgesics as endorphins by showing that the analgesic state could be abolished by administration of drugs that block effects of narcotics, such as Narcan.

The second noteworthy finding from Professor Wiertelak's experiment was observed following several days of repeatedly exposing the rats to the stressful stimulus (a series of shocks). Before long, the testing context itself elicited analgesia; Eric didn't need to shock the rats for them to start producing endorphins. The rats quickly figured out that the experimental room predicted danger, and prepared by making and releasing opioids ahead of time.

So far I've only described the first half of Professor Wiertelak's findings, so bear with me because it gets even more interesting. Some rats undergoing this protocol were shown a flash of light immediately following the last shock each day. In the same way that the experimental context predicted shock and stress, the light came to signal safety. Soon, the light began to reverse the rats' analgesia so that their pain sensitivity immediately returned to normal. Eric surmised that the safety signal led to the release of anti-opiates, and to prove this, he administered morphine to the rats before flashing the light. Within a *few seconds* of turning on the light predicting safety, the effects of morphine were abolished.

The half-life of morphine (the time it takes for blood levels of the drug to drop by 50 percent, due in this and most cases to metabolism by the liver) is over an hour, so the natural dissipation of morphine effects is nowhere near as fast as demonstrated in Eric's rats. Instead, realizing that they were "safe" must have led to a compensatory release of anti-opioids—a fabulous example of the *b process*. Earlier studies, by many researchers, had indicated that opiate tolerance and dependence involved an increase in anti-opiates. Eric added to this literature by showing that cues in the environment could turn on and off pain sensitivity by causing release of different neurotransmitters. One of my favorite stories concerning the neural modulation of pain comes from a student who managed to play the last few minutes of his school's championship soccer game with a cracked tibia and then to celebrate the close victory, all without experiencing any discomfort. It was only when he got into the family van to head home after the match that he suddenly became aware of excruciating pain. Mom and Dad were his safety signal. It's good news for our survival that pain sensitivity can be fine-tuned to the specifics of our situation, but bad news if you're seeking "free lunch" from a poppy plant.

In contrast to our other senses, pain is especially critical to our survival, and the sense is more like an individualistic lens that can open and close gates of sensory experience. For instance, blind, deaf, or anosmic people (the last are those with no sense of smell) are all likely to live a normal life span, but this is not the case for those who are born with a congenital insensitivity to pain who almost invariably die young, from complications following an injury.

Moreover, simply snipping a pair of cranial nerves could quickly render someone blind, deaf, or anosmic—the pathways are relatively simple, discrete, and well characterized. Pain is processed redundantly and diffusely, and there is simply no surgical intervention to relieve chronic pain (as many medical doctors and their patients know too well). Instead, pain recruits overlapping pathways and circuits throughout the body and brain and, along with a rich neurochemistry of opioids and antiopiates, portends the critical nature of pain for our survival.

Like Eric's rats, humans are expert at associating coincidences in the environment. We do so automatically, many times a day, throughout our lives. Effects of drugs are no exception; they are quickly associated with any and all information that predicts the effects are coming. Our reaction, though, is not the same as the reaction to the expected stimulus, but rather the opposite. Pavlov's dogs salivated at both food and the bell associated with mealtime. But if a drug makes your mouth water, the cues associated with the drug would give you cotton mouth instead. This apparent contradiction is understood by appreciating whether or not a stimulus acts directly on the CNS and recruits homeostatic processes. A drug does. Dinner does not.

Recipe for Misery

During my postdoc in Oregon, I briefly shared an office with a new dentist who, judging by the action his telephone received, was rather a popular fellow. He'd somehow gotten a reputation for being liberal with his prescription pad and as a result was harassed practically nonstop. I don't think he was at all cavalier about enabling addicts but simply gullible in his inability to recognize and defend against their persistence and determination. He'd try to plead and reason with "patients" while they came up with creative excuses for more pills. I remember more than one case of a person having all the teeth in his head removed, one at a time over several months, because each extraction warranted a fresh bottle of pills. My office mate noted with resignation (before changing buildings and phone numbers) that there was no objective way to assess the validity of a patient's claim of toothache, and at least when the last tooth was extracted the person would finally stop calling.

What desperation could lead a person to sacrifice the teeth in his mouth? Anti-opiates are at least partly to blame. Research has demonstrated that anti-opiates contribute to addiction as a major source of sickness and misery in opiate addicts. Dozens of peptides (short chains of amino acids) with anti-opiate properties have been identified. Some of the better known of these are dynorphin, orphanin FQ, cholecystokinin, and NPFF, all of which may facilitate adaptation and contribute to tolerance, dependence, and craving. Still, they don't account for the breadth of opiate addiction on their own. Scientists have identified several other forms of adaptation that contribute: some implicate the brain's immune system; many others involve compensatory changes inside individual brain cells. Although the number of opiate receptors isn't dramatically decreased in a chronic narcotic user (the way CB_1 receptors decrease in marijuana smokers), the ability of opiates to affect intracellular signaling is compromised with frequent use, so the receptors are downregulated in effectiveness if not in number.

But the anti-opiate system is the cruelest. Because an addict's nervous system is regularly flooded with compounds that produce euphoria, the anti-opiate system ramps up to *create* pain so that the net effect is something like normal sensation. This opposing anti-opiate system can be turned on by safety, or by the expectation of safety after danger passes, but it's likely that there is no more effective way to activate anti-opiate processes than through regular exposure to opiates, which must be like a perfect nail to these finely evolved hammers.

Furthermore, cues that predict drug use lead to activation of the anti-opiate system, too. Seeing a spoon in a bathroom, for instance, is enough to cause chills and craving in any mainline opiate user, even if they haven't picked up for years. In general, the more extensive one's using experience is, the more triggers one is likely to have. Stress is an especially potent cue because it leads to a "taste" of actual opioid activity, but other subtler factors—like time, place, people, money, and music—have the same consequence: anti-opiate-induced craving and physical and psychological symptoms associated with withdrawal. (To get a comprehensive idea of anti-opiate effects, scan the second column in the table on p. 76.)

This is to say that opiate addiction (like all addiction) is to some degree contextual. Such a point was made most strongly in recent history by a large group of U.S. veterans of the Vietnam War. Up to 20 percent of these troops sought escape by taking narcotics that were readily available in Southeast Asia. Congress had some warning of the pending problem as the troops were scheduled to return home at the end of the war, and national hearings were held by the Nixon administration to figure out what to do. It was decided that soldiers who tested positive would be detoxed overseas and carefully tracked upon their return. This strategy turned out to be fortuitous because the dramatically different context at home seemed to powerfully contribute to successful abstinence. In fact, only about 5 percent of the soldiers addicted in Vietnam ended up relapsing (compared with about 90 percent of people addicted and treated here). We can presume that exposure to a context similar to that experienced in Nam—such as dense, humid jungle or gunfire—might have produced a more typical rate of relapse.

Paying the Piper

The brain adapts to all exogenous chemicals that alter its activity, but the degree of tolerance, dependence, and craving in opiate users is legend—stronger than for almost every other drug. Adaptations that underlie opiate addiction, including the production of anti-opiates, begin during the very first administration (this is true of all drugs) and rapidly gain strength with use. The strength of these opponent processes may be so robust because the sensation of pain is so critical for survival.

As a result, with time, a dose that initially worked well will hardly produce any effect at all, and in order to realize the same experience, you'd have to take more. Of course, if you increase your dose, then the adaptation will be even greater to meet the bigger challenge. This means you'll have to take more again. Thus, the romance is no longer hot when your lover is present, but when your lover is absent your body and mind are overcome with suffering—all as a result of the nervous system's profound adaptation. Naturally, this leads to craving, because anything is better than the excruciating desolation of abstinence.

Opiate tolerance is mind-bogglingly robust. Addicts can administer upwards of 150 *times* the dose that would be lethal to naive users and, even so, just feel "right" but not really high. In laboratory studies, it takes fully tolerant animals a "drug holiday" of nearly six days in order to regain just half of the intrinsic sensitivity to morphine that will get them high (no need to point out that half a high is hardly going to satisfy). In contrast, the half-life associated with the return of sensitivity to nicotine is about half an hour, and complete recovery and resensitization occur when doses of this drug are separated by only three hours. Full opiate recovery is likely to take weeks or months, which is the primary reason it is so hard for addicts to kick.

By definition, people are dependent on a drug when they experience withdrawal symptoms in its absence. Maintaining an opiate habit is expensive and time-consuming, and despite all the resources going toward scoring and using, the drug doesn't really work because of tolerance. So, many addicts attempt to quit, and when they do, they suffer with a constellation of withdrawal symptoms exactly opposite to the acute effects of the drug. In addition to several leaking orifices, someone withdrawing from opiates will be unable to either be still or rest.

OPIATE EFFECTS	WITHDRAWAL SYMPTOMS
Analgesia	Pain
Respiratory depression	Panting and yawning
Euphoria	Irritability and dysphoria
Relaxation and sleep	Restlessness and insomnia
Tranquilization	Fearfulness and hostility
Decreased blood pressure	Increased blood pressure
Constipation	Diarrhea
Pupil constriction	Pupil dilation
Decreased core temperature	Increased core temperature
Dried secretions	Tearing and runny nose
Reduced sex drive	Spontaneous orgasm
Flushed and warm skin	Chilliness and goose bumps

One way to understand the dilemma of the opiate user is to recognize that because there are no free lunches, the benefits that drugs confer will have to be paid back. In principle, moments of superb contentment demand an equal and opposite experience of distress; the benefit of euphoria will create a debt of dysphoria; and trying to avoid this unpleasant state by taking more drug will just increase what you owe. In practice, the depth and extent of the withdrawal period is in direct proportion to the duration and intensity of the drug bathing the brain. Just as the first exposure is "best," likewise, the first time someone tries to get clean is the easiest, and easier still if the period of using was of short duration. Easier maybe, but this would only be known in retrospect. Any experience of kicking will feel like the antithesis of our desire. But medicating it will not only put off the misery but strengthen it for next time.

Until the past few years, most career addicts were in their forties or fifties and after so many years of pillowing through life were frankly not expected to ever get clean. Methadone was promoted as a substitute solution for these people who, with daily administration of this drug in a clinical setting, could exist in a liminal state of neither well nor sick. Methadone acts as a substitute opiate—one that is orally absorbed and has an especially long half-life. Drinking a daily "cocktail" at the clinic prevents withdrawal (as well as antisocial activities that help keep withdrawal at bay, like stealing and shooting up in public places), and because the drug is so cheap, it's been seen as of great benefit—though likely less to the addicts than to members of their communities.

Recently, however, methadone has been used in younger and younger addicts. This is especially tragic, if not unethical, from both a neurobiological and a social perspective. Because methadone is such a long-lasting opiate, when prescribed with the clinical goal of keeping the brain soaked in the stuff to stave off withdrawal, it produces an immense addiction. This drug is even harder to kick than heroin; the latter is hell, but for a relatively short time. Therefore, to prescribe a drug like this to people barely out of their teens is to condone "maintenance" that is in some ways a life sentence akin to housing the mentally ill in the back wards of state institutions: they'll be less trouble for the rest of us, but unlikely to have much of a life.

A better strategy from a neurological perspective might be to employ the opposite tack. Instead of bathing the cells in opiates for long periods, knock them over the head with a big dose of anti-opiates! Giving anti-opiates should induce the brain to maintain homeostasis by upregulating, or at least normalizing, its opioid system. This has in fact been tried and in some ways works like a charm. Here's how it goes: you check into a hospital, receive general anesthesia (the reason for this will be clear momentarily), and take a whopping dose of Narcan. This drug occupies all of the same sites opiates do but doesn't activate them. If Narcan is administered to unsedated addicts who haven't been using, they will come *unglued*—instantaneously experiencing the throes of withdrawal. However, if they are anesthetized while their brain is bathed with high doses of the drug, then the cells adapt back to their naive state in fairly short order.

Sounds terrific, right? Unfortunately, it doesn't take long for some users, once awakened, to recognize their nascent state and take advantage by checking out of the hospital to score. Another problem with this strategy is that it only works for those who can afford it—like the rock star who enjoyed his hiatus about every other month at the elite psychiatric hospital in South Florida where I worked for a summer. On the other hand, a former stripper I know who became a rocket scientist after getting clean argued that remembering the punishing throes of withdrawal helped her remain abstinent after kicking and that if she'd been able to sleep through this misery, she might never have been so motivated.

A more enlightened and democratic approach falls almost exactly in the middle of these extremes. Suboxone is a combination of a Narcan-like drug and an opiate drug called buprenorphine. Buprenorphine doesn't have much street appeal for the same reason it's a good choice here: although it occupies the same places in the brain as opiate drugs, it doesn't do as good a job and therefore it is much less rewarding than its abused counterparts. However, the effects are potent enough to reduce symptoms of withdrawal, including craving, and to allow addicts to sleep. It's less stigmatizing than methadone, but even more important, under a doctor's supervision, it won't make the addiction stronger. For someone motivated to get clean, this could provide a sound start. If the dose is tapered over time, it's likely to afford the best shot at a life free from opiate addiction.

The bottom line for opiate users, and the bottom line of this book, is that there can never be enough drug. Because of the brain's tremendous capacity to adapt, it's impossible for a regular user to get high, and the best a voracious appetite for more drug can hope to accomplish is to stave off withdrawal. This situation is best recognized as a dead end.

5

The Sledgehammer: Alcohol

I stood to my feet
in the midst of the cosmos,
appearing outwardly in flesh.
I discovered that all were drunk
and none were thirsty,
and my soul ached for
the children of humanity.
For their hearts are blind
and they cannot see from within.
They have come into the cosmos empty,
and they are leaving it empty.
At the moment you are inebriated,
but free from the effects of wine,
you too may turn and stand.

—Logion 28, *The Gospel of Thomas: Wisdom*
of the Twin (translated by Lynn C. Bauman)

A Defense

Almost exactly seven years after getting clean and sober, I exited
the cramped room where I'd spent hours defending my dissertation before a committee of expert scientists. My thesis sought
to explain the mechanisms responsible for the observation that
morphine tolerance is higher in familiar contexts than in novel

ones. My studies helped build the case that the more we anticipate morphine effects, the more likely our nervous system is to
recruit natural anti-opiates. As I departed the seminar room
with a mixture of feelings—from relief and exhaustion to pride
and elation—I was greeted by several fellow graduate students
loitering in the hallway waiting to hear the news and, hopefully,
to congratulate me. Frank was the first to give me a perfunctory
slap on the back, along with a stiff smile. He looked a little off,
and when I asked what was the matter, he blurted right out that
none of the group knew how to celebrate with me because it was
convention that the occasion be commemorated with a champagne toast and I didn't drink.

My life had changed 180 degrees. Not only did I have a shiny
new Ph.D., but I was able to look people in the eye and feed my
respectable habits without committing crimes. I'd wake up
every morning feeling clean and rested, knowing where I was
and more or less what my day would hold—a state so precious
that everyone should be so fortunate. Things were so much better for me that I wish I had laughed easily and suggested cup-
cakes or a hike on the Flatirons. But instead my first thought
after Frank's awkward reminder was "Damn right! I've busted
my ass all these years and deserve a drink!" It may be hard
for any sane person to appreciate the depth of self-pity I felt
because I couldn't toast the accomplishment in plastic cups
with my fellows.

Social convention is pickled in the intoxicating juice of alcohol. In 1839, an English traveler named Frederick Marryat noted
in his diary that American practice was "if you meet, you drink; if
you part, you drink; if you make acquaintance, you drink; if you
close a bargain, you drink; they quarrel in their drink, and they
make it up with a drink. They drink, because it is hot; they drink,
because it is cold."[1] This custom certainly hasn't diminished in

the past couple of centuries, and it presents a tremendous challenge to recovery. I don't suppose those refusing cocaine or even marijuana encounter the mix of incredulity and pity that those of us refusing alcohol regularly experience. Well-meaning hosts, reflecting a strong social consensus, persist despite repeated refusals by offering more and more options or insisting we have "just one." Advertising promotions, made-to-order drinking occasions, and the pervasive presence of the drug itself are all impossible to avoid and present a thought-provoking paradox.

If alcohol and other drug addictions were rare events, unlikely except for a few tragic cases, it would be one thing. But in the face of superabundant examples proximal, ubiquitous, and concrete, as well as our own family wounds concerning the stuff, our deep collective denial is strange. The manic insistence on ignoring the obvious is reminiscent of cigarette commercials I grew up watching. The juxtaposition of youthful athleticism with a nicotine habit seemed as odd to me as a child as the insistence today that alcohol somehow makes everything sexier and livelier. I still remember one commercial in particular that showed a group of gorgeously tanned young adults whitewater rafting down a rugged canyon as they promoted a popular menthol brand. Really? Smoking while rafting?

This incongruity is thoroughly pervasive. We always kick off the annual meeting of the Research Society on Alcoholism, where I recently received my twenty-five-year membership pin, with a reception. Free drink tickets—two per person, just right for the social drinker—are offered to everyone, and the drug flows freely (because you can pay cash when your tickets run out). This doesn't seem unusual; after all, there's hardly a time or place where alcohol isn't expected, but what strikes me is the stark contrast in options. Those who imbibe have a surfeit of tasty-looking possibilities (I realize that they may seem especially so to me, but this is my point rather than beside it), while the few of us there who don't drink are offered soda or water. Water is my drink of choice now, but can't it at least be good water? And why no freshly squeezed juices or other yummy options? After all, this is a group of experts on alcoholism!

The bipolar practice of pitying addicts while at the same time greasing virtually every social interaction with an obscene amount and variety of booze seems heartless if not mindless. It's also exclusionary—as if the only truly comfortable place for people who can't handle their drink were under a bridge. I can certainly understand that my not drinking may make some people uncomfortable. Perhaps it seems I'm reneging on the grand social contract to blur assessment as people let off steam. It is true that it is sometimes hard to be around a group of people drinking socially, but not because I'm judging their consumption or tendency to disclose in a way that doesn't comport with what I know of their sober selves. Rather, it can be lonely.

I am also particularly curious about the general practice of celebrating peak experiences with a sedative. I understand that it is easy to be overwhelmed by strong emotions, and I appreciate the desire to evade stark reality, but still, it seems odd that we drink and use to permit or enhance strong feelings as well as to mute them. I've been to others' graduations, countless weddings, sporting events, or similar festivities where the norm is to celebrate by dimming the lights. Though the appeal is understandable—something like sleeping through a child's birth—as someone who has tried it both ways, I'm a fan of showing up. True, at times life can be awful, disappointing, terrifying, or mind-numbingly tedious. But just the same, there is the frequent possibility of being overcome with joy, gratitude, or delight. In short, it is likely impossible to tamp down terror without also leveling pleasure. As Socrates noted, and many appreciate, sorrow and joy depend on each other; I prefer the roller coaster to the train.

Musings like these led me to consider other options for celebrating my dissertation defense. Instead of getting blotto, I found an inexpensive plane ticket and spent seven weeks in the South Pacific—with a backpack and a sense of accomplishment, alone except for people I met along the way. What a poor substitute even a cellar full of champagne would have been for kayaking in Milford Sound, completing my open dive certification on the Great Barrier Reef, and being proposed to by a Fijian chief!

Make It Stop, Please!

We use drugs in large part because of their pleasurable effects, a form of what scientists call positive reinforcement. There is a high correlation between a drug's addictive liability and its capacity to induce dopamine-mediated positive reinforcement. But the drive to experience good feelings is not sufficient to account fully for the liability toward abuse, especially alcohol abuse. People also take drugs in order to reduce unpleasant feelings. This tendency is called negative reinforcement, and the motivation it provides is critical.

Alcohol and other downers are negatively reinforcing in part because they reduce anxiety; opiates are so compelling because they reduce suffering; stimulants because they reduce boredom. Moreover, because alcohol reduces anxiety, this drug will be more reinforcing to those who are naturally anxious than to those who are not, increasing the risk of regular drinking in such individuals. There is good evidence that those of us who are naturally inclined toward any of these predisposing states are more likely to abuse the "complementary" substance.

However, because the brain adapts to the neural changes

wrought by any drug, the effects of chronic exposure are going to undermine any attempts at self-medication. Alas, if someone finds alcohol especially rewarding because of an inherited tendency toward anxiety and she imbibes frequently, she'll become increasingly anxious and require more drug.

Both positive and negative reinforcements are balanced in practice by what might be called the punishing aspects of drug use, and although punishment is generally less effective in shaping behavior than is reinforcement, it also comes in two forms that can play a role in addiction.

Positive punishment stems from unpleasant consequences that decrease the likelihood of subsequent use. Effects such as vomiting or having a hangover and consequences such as fines and public admonitions may serve to decrease a propensity for regular use.

The first drug prescribed specifically to treat alcoholics was based on the premise of positive punishment. Antabuse interferes with the metabolism of alcohol and leads to a buildup of acetaldehyde, which is toxic. This metabolite produces uncomfortable physiological effects including flushing, sweating, and irregular heartbeat. Though it is still used to some benefit by highly motivated individuals, forty years of research have largely confirmed what most parents and pet owners already know: in general, punishment is not an especially effective way to change behavior.

Some people live as if permanently taking Antabuse because of a natural deficiency in the enzyme that metabolizes acetaldehyde, caused by a common gene variation. These mutations are fairly rare in those with European descent but present in about half of northeast Asians. Within an hour after consuming alcohol, such people experience allergic-like reactions to the drug, including facial flushing, hives, and shortness of breath. Not surprisingly, this mutation decreases the tendency toward excessive drinking; however, it doesn't totally prevent alcoholism, demonstrating the limited efficacy of punishment on behavior. Other people have deficiencies in the primary enzyme that is responsible for metabolizing nicotine, and for these smokers the concentration of the drug in the blood gets higher and stays high longer. Because too much of this drug is also unpleasant, these people are less likely to smoke, and when they do, they are more likely to successfully quit. Chalk one up for positive punishment.

Negative punishment occurs as things we find pleasurable are taken away as a result of our behavior. For example, we might lose our jobs, our self-respect, deplete our bank accounts, or alienate our families. Once again, courts and prisons are full of people for whom this strategy has failed. Somehow the threat of losing everything is usually insufficient for addicts inclined to pick up. For some others, though, negative punishment may deter the development of regular use, and thus help prevent the slide into addiction. Marijuana produces notoriously varied and subjective effects, including a tendency toward sleepiness in some people, although we don't yet know why. However, because passing out is no way to "party," they seem to be deterred from regular pot smoking.

My friend Levi was a wonderful human being but also a chronic alcoholic. Because he and his wife could not stop drinking, they lost custody of all six of their children, and when I knew them, they were heartbroken and homeless, living on the streets of Boulder, Colorado. Levi wanted to stop drinking but simply couldn't manage to string together more than a couple of days sober. At the time, you couldn't purchase alcohol in the city limits on Sunday, and perhaps because he wasn't much of a planner, he came up with a solution he called "White Lightning." He'd use a can opener to puncture a hole toward the bottom of Aqua Net hairspray and consume the "cocktail" quickly, before gagging on the taste. He also took Antabuse, but neither did that seem to slow him down. He'd feel ill and look terrible but drink right through a toxic state, explaining that his brain needed alcohol whether his body liked it or not. Despite his warm heart and both types of punishment, he froze to death one night while passed out on the banks of Boulder Creek.

We might assume that Levi had a high tolerance for punishment, as in fact do most addicts, which is part of the reason that punitive treatment hasn't had much impact. It is also true that dramatic changes in the balance of these four forces—positive and negative reinforcement and positive and negative punishment—occur with regular use in a way that makes addiction more likely. In particular, we rapidly form a tolerance to positive reinforcing effects, while the negatively reinforcing effects typically become stronger as users use more to stave off symptoms associated with withdrawal.

In other words, addicts may be those who are especially charmed by the quality of carrots and immune to the beating of sticks, as any municipal court could attest.

Actions

It might seem that alcohol would be straightforward to research and understand. There's hardly a person on the planet not familiar with the drug, and the molecule itself is beguilingly simple, made from not much more than a couple of carbon atoms. Ethyl alcohol, or ethanol, the alcohol we drink, is readily produced by fermentation, which occurs naturally when sugar comes into contact with yeast and water. Rotting fruit and wet grain were probably the conduits for our ancestors' first tastes, but it didn't take long for intentional brewing to ensure a steady supply—beginning at least eleven thousand years ago. Because the process of fermentation is so simple, it has been discovered and exploited by virtually every human culture.

C_2H_5OH, the ethanol molecule

In some times and places, natural alcoholic beverages were used as the primary drink for all citizens, but it has also been employed as medicine or as part of a social or religious ceremony. For instance, the Aztec Native Americans reserved pulque, a traditional beverage made from the sap of the agave plant, for sacred use, except that people older than seventy could drink it as often as they wished. In India, *sura* brewed from rice, wheat, sugar, and fruits has been popular for millennia, along with an admonition against excessive consumption.

Yeasts are living microorganisms that can't survive in alcohol conditions above 10–15 percent, so the natural synthesis of alcohol produces a relatively low-concentration beverage. Even today, self-synthesizing products like beer and wine must be consumed in fairly large quantities to produce desired effects, making it somewhat less likely for people to use in excess. However, the discovery of distillation, probably by the ancient Greeks in the first century A.D., upped the ante significantly.

Distillation involves boiling the concoction to collect the alcohol, which evaporates first. Distilled spirits include a range of favorites such as whiskey, rum, vodka, and tequila, which have alcohol concentrations around 40–50 percent. Paradoxically, the simplicity of the ethanol molecule is what makes it so difficult to understand. Molecules of cocaine, THC, heroin, and ecstasy are much larger and more structurally complex, and therefore their sites of action in the brain are very specific. Alcohol is so small and wily its actions are hard to pin down. It's easy to imagine that there are many more places to park a skateboard than an airplane. Because the effect of a drug is dependent on this "parking" or "binding," and alcohol does this at multiple sites, its effects are also much less specific.

Some of it is metabolized in the stomach, though more for men than for women due to sex differences in the amount of enzyme contained in the gastric fluid. Nonetheless, it diffuses out of the stomach at a rate that depends on how much food is there, and even what kind of food, heading straight for the liver. Normally, alcohol is degraded at a constant rate, in contrast to other drugs whose metabolism depends on their concentration, and the drug reaches equilibrium in the blood and brain in less than an hour. This "first pass" metabolism, indeed all alcohol metabolism, is highly variable among people, with efficiency especially tied to genetics, drinking and other drug history, and age. For most people, liver enzymes can take care of a little over a drink an hour as the drug is first converted to acetaldehyde, then to vinegar, and finally to carbon dioxide and water.

When any drug has an effect, it's due to the drug's chemical actions on brain structures. For most drugs of abuse, we know precisely which structures are modified, and this gives us a really good start to understanding how they make us feel the way they do. Cocaine blocks a protein that recycles dopamine, and because dopamine hangs around longer than usual, we feel euphoric and energized. For alcohol, the target(s) are not as clear, which is to say that the mechanisms of drunkenness are still being worked out.

We know this much: the transcendent sense I felt in a friend's basement as I guzzled wine was the result of sundry molecular effects. My sense of ease was likely due to the drug's foremost neural consequence: facilitating GABA neurotransmission. GABA is one of the most prevalent neurotransmitters and *the* primary inhibitory neurotransmitter in the brain. Because GABA-mediated inhibition is enhanced by alcohol, neural activity slows down. At moderate doses this reduces anxiety, but at higher concentrations it produces sedation and eventually sleep (sometimes known as passing out). Enhancing activity at GABA synapses likely made me feel very relaxed.

Alcohol also reduces activity at glutamate receptors. Glutamate happens to be the primary excitatory neurotransmitter, so this plus GABA inhibition really tamps down the electrical activity of neurons. Glutamate is also critical for forming new memories, and if I had blacked out that day (that is, forgotten chunks of experience), it likely would have been from alcohol's ability to impede glutamate's activity. Because glutamate and GABA are so prevalent, alcohol slows neural activity throughout the brain, not just in a few pathways, explaining the drug's global effects on cognition, emotion, memory, and movement.

As with all addictive drugs, alcohol produces rapid subjective changes in affect that are typical of mesolimbic activation, including a sense of pleasure and possibility. In alcohol's case, this effect is thought to reflect activation of opioid receptors by endogenous opioids, which then lead to dopamine release.

The pharmacological mishmash includes a slew of other effects, and the relationship between these chemical interactions and what we experience is less well understood. For example, alcohol also slows neural activity by impeding neurotransmitter release through its actions on calcium channels. Calcium is a necessary catalyst for exocytosis—the process by which synaptic vesicles release neurotransmitters into the cleft between neurons—so because the chemical communication between cells is impeded, normal messages may not be sent, perhaps contributing to confusion or difficulties with speech or other movements. At high concentrations, alcohol may also have general effects on the physical integrity of brain cells. Neuron membranes are basically made of fat. Bathing them in alcohol causes the membranes to become more and more fluid, and as the cell structure is compromised, so is the ability of neurons to conduct information—leading to stupor or unconsciousness. The drug can also interact with a particular type of serotonin receptor as well as acetylcholine receptors, perhaps impacting mood and cognition. No wonder we've had such a hard time clarifying its actions in the brain. Compared with virtually every other drug of abuse, which typically interacts in a very specific way with only a single neural substrate, alcohol is so promiscuous it's hard to pin down how each of its chemical kisses contributes to the intoxicating effects we experience.

In addition to all of the classic neurotransmitter interactions just described, alcohol interacts with scores of peptides. There are hundreds of peptide transmitter systems—each a topic of intense research. The purpose of my drilling down on one, beta-endorphin, besides sharing a topic of my own research, is to illustrate the breadth and depth of research inquiry into this simple yet complicated drug.

We have long known that alcohol use rapidly leads to the synthesis and release of beta-endorphin, a string of thirty-one amino acids that is thought to contribute to the drug's euphoric and relaxing effects by increasing mesolimbic dopamine levels and inhibiting the "fight or flight" response. This system is the target of one of the pharmaceutical strategies to combat alcohol abuse, naltrexone, a longer-acting and orally available cousin of naloxone, which is marketed as Narcan. Both naltrexone and naloxone firmly park on opioid receptors but don't activate them. (Thus they are called opioid antagonists.) Naltrexone, marketed as ReVia and Vivitrol, occupies these sites for relatively long periods so that when a person drinks alcohol, any endorphin activity is rendered moot. Narcan/naloxone doesn't hang around as long but effectively reverses an opiate overdose by fitting even better than opiates do into the "parking" spot and therefore kicking them out. My interest in this peptide was piqued many years ago when I learned of a series of studies spearheaded by Christina Gianoulakis at McGill University. She and others had seen differences in the natural activity of beta-endorphin between those at high and those at low risk for excessive alcohol consumption. Over the years, a wealth of data from studies on twins had demonstrated that about 50–60 percent of the risk for alcoholism came from inherited factors.[2] And those who have a positive family history for alcoholism are three to five times more likely to develop the disease than those without such a background,[3] though the particular genes responsible remain largely unknown. Dr. Gianoulakis and her colleagues showed that high-risk individuals have about half as much beta-endorphin in their blood as those at low genetic risk;[4] Jan Froehlich and her colleagues then showed that these levels come largely from our parents.[5] But most interesting to me was the fact that alcohol was able to remedy this natural deficit especially in those who inherit a high risk for excessive drinking and, at higher doses, produce a surfeit of the peptide.[6]

Because beta-endorphin contributes to a sense of well-being

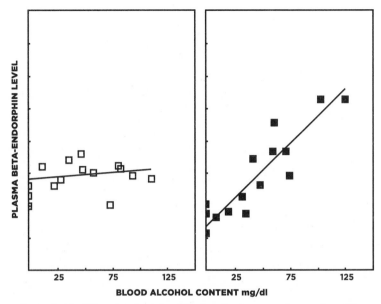

The heritable differences in endorphin signaling between those at low risk (left) and high risk (right) for alcohol abuse. Data adapted from Gianoulakis et al., 1989.

by soothing stress and facilitating social affiliation, those of us with naturally low levels may experience less sense of safety and connection, even as children, on a day-to-day basis. That is, until John Barleycorn is invited to the party! Data such as these suggest that some of us are especially likely to find alcohol reinforcing because we can use it to medicate an innate opioid deficiency. Perhaps the "hole in my soul" I felt finally filled in my friend's basement was nothing more than a flood of endorphins at last quenching destitute receptors.

Effects

Alcohol is a neurological sledgehammer. By acting throughout the brain to influence a multitude of targets, the drug affects virtually all aspects of neural functioning. One or two drinks help to blur the edges, and a reduction in anxiety promotes relaxation. But with a few more drinks, a person loses inhibitions as cortical monitoring is shut down and subcortical, "emotional" regions are freed from normal constraints. As one approaches the legal limit for alcohol in the blood, behavior is sedated, and speech and coordination are impaired. Still more drinking and the person might lose consciousness. These effects are what justify alcohol's classification as a sedative-hypnotic.

Most drugs are effective in the milligram range, but alcohol begins to produce these subjective effects only after almost a hundred times a typical drug dose is administered. Potency doesn't really matter for practical purposes, though, especially because we've come up with so many tasty ways to use a "spoonful of sugar to make the medicine go down," and it's perfectly legal to consume in most settings. As the concentration in the blood and brain increases, judgment is impaired and motor skills decline while risky behavior increases, along with memory and concentration problems, emotional volatility, loss of coordination, including slurred speech, and confusion. Finally, nausea rises and vomiting begins as the area postrema, otherwise known as the brain's vomit center, reflexively works to expel the poison. Eventually, the drinker could fall into a coma. If intoxication occurs very rapidly—for instance, by guzzling high-potency beverages on an empty stomach—it's possible for the anesthetic effects to occur before the vomit reflex is engaged. In this case, as the brain is shut down, it's possible to die from overdose.

All of the neurochemical actions I've described are neural responses to alcohol; in other words, they represent many of the drug's *a processes,* which are readily produced in naive or irregular users. But of course, with chronic exposure, each of these elicits a complementary *b process* as the brain adapts in order to maintain physiological equilibrium. GABA systems become less sensitive and glutamate more sensitive, making the brain more active in the absence of the drug and producing much of the neuroexcitability that underlies dangerous physical symptoms of alcoholic withdrawal, including seizures. Regular drinkers also see a downregulation of endorphin synthesis, and this likely contributes to a general malaise experienced during early abstinence. Naturally, these changes undermine the very effects that the drinker is seeking.

The consequences of intoxication can go well beyond individual brains. For example, impaired judgment can result in inappropriate sexual behavior, sexually transmitted infections, and unwanted pregnancies. It can also contribute to sexual assault, rape, and sexual trauma. Nearly 700,000 students a year in the United States between the ages of eighteen and twenty-four are assaulted by another student who has been drinking. In addition, about a third of all traffic-related fatalities in the United States are related to alcohol intoxication, and numerous studies have found a high correlation between substance use and intimate partner violence.

Excessive, chronic drinking leads to cardiovascular problems including stroke and high blood pressure; liver problems such as steatosis (fatty liver), alcoholic hepatitis, fibrosis, and cirrhosis; pancreatitis; and increased risk of various cancers (including of the mouth, esophagus, larynx, pharynx, breast, liver, colon, and rectum). But even moderate drinking is harmful. A recent study evaluated the effects of drinking in over half a million people around the world and found that even one drink a day is associated with a number of diseases (including cancers and cardiovascular issues) that lead to premature death.[7] The more people drank, the worse the outcome: about two drinks a day shaves a year or two off the life span, and reduced intake increases life expectancy. In addition, alcohol use during pregnancy can lead to a wide range of disabilities in children, the most severe of which is fetal alcohol syndrome, characterized by intellectual disabilities, speech and language delays, poor social skills, and sometimes facial deformities.

Despite these grim outcomes, it seems that we can neither get enough of the drug nor get it fast enough. In the United States, more than a quarter of people over eighteen reported that they engaged in binge drinking during the previous month. This pattern is even more prevalent among college students, nearly 40 percent of whom reported binge drinking in the previous month. Whether cause or effect, about half of these students (20 percent) meet the criteria for an alcohol use disorder, and 25 percent report academic consequences from drinking. Binge drinking is risky for anyone, but particularly for those whose brains are still developing. The impact of high alcohol concentrations during this "plastic" period leads to lasting alterations in brain structure and function and is more likely to result in an alcohol use disorder. The converse is also true: one of the most effective ways to curtail the risk of addiction is to avoid intoxication during periods of rapid brain development. People who begin drinking in their early teens, as I did, are at least four times more likely to eventually meet the criteria for an alcohol use disorder. In fact, the lifetime risk for substance abuse and dependence decreases about 5 percent with each additional year between ages thirteen and twenty-one.[8] Yet young people are especially prone to binge drinking in part because they are neurobiologically primed to seek and appreciate novel and high-risk experiences. Though their parents may not appreciate it, for adolescents these tendencies are well timed to promote the development of adult goals and identity formation.

Binge drinking, defined for females as more than four drinks within two hours, and for males more than five, is enough to raise blood concentrations above the legal threshold to operate an automobile. The dosage difference between the sexes is due to the fact that it takes less alcohol for women to achieve the same blood concentrations as men. This is due to differences in the concentration of the ALDH enzyme found in the gut, mentioned above, as well as sex differences in the proportion of body fat. A male typically has more blood than an equally weighted female because women have a higher proportion of body fat, and fat requires less blood than muscle does. Lower blood volume and slower metabolism may also partly explain the steeper dive in women alcoholics who more quickly progress to organ damage, disordered use, and death from drinking.

Alcohol's effects are also dependent on environmental factors. For instance, whether the drug produces more sedation or euphoria depends in part on whether drinking occurs while consoling oneself after getting fired or celebrating a promotion. There is great cultural variation, too, in the ways people express their intoxication. The pub scene might look very different in Tokyo, Belfast, and Copenhagen, because social mores shape behavior, to an extent that might make it hard for an alien visitor to accept that we were all experiencing the same molecule. And on an individual basis, differences in brain chemistry can produce a different balance of pleasurable and aversive effects. Stimulant drugs like cocaine and amphetamine produce effects that are much more universal, in part because their actions in the brain are so precise.

As a rule, sedation is not as much enjoyed as stimulation, which is why, despite its popularity, alcohol is not as addictive as are some other drugs. Over 85 percent of the world's adults drink, but only about one-tenth of these develop a problem.

Also, even though the ethanol in all alcoholic beverages is the same molecule, different beverages contain different congeners or impurities from the distillation process, often connected to the source—tequila has more congeners than vodka—that can affect the experience of intoxication and withdrawal (that is, they can produce a worse hangover).

Consequences

All behavior, including addiction, is in some ways context dependent. My using was situated in the last quarter of the twentieth century, socially and culturally very different from the new millennium. I'm not sure how much differently we drank—perhaps the names and the games have changed—but certainly the consequences varied. For example, one evening, when I was only fifteen or sixteen and in possession of a new driving permit, I decided to practice my skills and get out of the house after supper. It's hard to imagine now, because things have swung so much the other way, but heading east toward the ocean, I breezed through a red light toking on a joint with a beer between my legs. As smoke billowed out the window, the policeman who pulled me over gaped briefly with a mixture of concern and surprise before admonishing me to "be careful"! Another time a girlfriend and I were flagged over as we weaved down Dixie Highway in the wee hours of the morning and were only given a warning after we assured the officer we were able to drive home safely. I doubt there are many places in the United States where this would happen today.

While the consequences have generally gotten stricter, the per capita consumption both here and worldwide has been rising fairly steeply since my heyday. Excessive use of alcohol now results in about 3.3 million deaths around the world each year.[9] In Russia and its former satellite states, one in five male deaths is caused by drinking. And in the United States during the period between 2006 and 2010, excessive alcohol use was responsible for close to 90,000 deaths a year, including one in ten deaths among adults aged twenty to sixty-four, translating to 2.5 million years of potential life lost. More than half of these deaths and three-quarters of the years of potential life lost were due to binge drinking.

Alcohol use also substantially contributes to automobile accidents, domestic abuse, and other forms of violence. Roughly a third of all visits to emergency rooms for injuries in 2016 were alcohol related. Given all this, it is perhaps surprising that alcohol is only the second most lethal drug—trailing not opiates as one might suspect after reading almost any newspaper or magazine but the other legal substance: tobacco. In fact, alcohol killed about twice as many people in 2016 as prescription opioids and heroin overdoses combined, and even this number would be almost three times higher if it included drunk-driving-related deaths.

Alcohol's low potency in the brain thus belies its disproportionate influence on human suffering: for a substantial minority (between 10 and 15 percent) and their communities, the consequences of alcohol addiction are devastating, and it's the third-largest cause of preventable death.[10] In fact, it's partly because it is such a small and slippery drug, able to influence all sorts of neural systems, and so readily produced, that it has such tremendous influence.

Alcohol has been such a huge part of our culture since we had culture that it can be nearly impossible to see the ways we all participate in the unsustainable epidemic of alcoholism. So we walk a fine line, glancing up at the scope of the battlefield, looking in the mirror at the ways we contribute, but mostly walking with our eyes cast down, perhaps as my colleague felt meeting me in the hallway after my successful dissertation defense.

What separated me from my colleague that day was not just the tradition of a champagne toast; it was the chasm between those who can and those who can't in a world that practically revolves around drinking. This wouldn't be so terrible except that so many of us are dying in plain sight as our neighbors, friends, and co-workers carry on blithely.

And the collective denial has real, rising implications. A further increase in drinking is actually good for some. Worldwide annual revenue from alcohol sales is about $150 billion. Diageo and Anheuser-Busch InBev are two of the leading global producers and have net profit margins of around 25 percent as they invest more in marketing than they do in payroll. In its 2013 annual report, Anheuser-Busch InBev articulated its goal to "create new occasions to share our products with consumers." This seems funny, because it obviously isn't creating the occasion, but rather the excuse to use an occasion for drinking. These businesses are well aware of psychological learning principles as they work to associate contexts with alcohol, noting that "insights have enabled us to create and position products for specific moments of consumption: enjoying a game or music event with friends, shifting toward a more relaxed mood after work, celebrating at a party or sharing a meal." Along similar lines, in 2014 the British Beer Alliance, a consortium of major British brewers, invested £10 million in the marketing campaign "There's a Beer for That," aiming to showcase "the variety of beer available in the UK and how these different styles fit perfectly a wide range of occasions."

Because even with new occasions there is presumably a limit to what existing markets can absorb, these and other large corporations have also focused on expanding sales by seeking new customers in previously fallow markets in low- and middle-income countries. They accomplish this by formulating cheap products for the mass market. For example, SABMiller, now a division of Anheuser-Busch InBev, offers Chibuku Shake-Shake across Africa. Chibuku was first brewed in the 1950s by a German brewer working in Zambia using sorghum, maize, and cassava. The drink is relatively unfiltered so that fermentation continues after packaging, often in cardboard cartons that have to be shaken to distribute particulates of starch, yeast, and plant germ—accounting for its fun name and cheap cost. Small plastic alcohol sachets are also increasingly common in many African countries. At the same time, Western brands are promoted to middle-class consumers in low-income countries as a status symbol. For example, Diageo claims its alcoholic apple drink Snapp provides African women with a beverage "more refined than beer, with cues of differentiation and sophistication." Similarly, there seem to be efforts to secure the next generations of consumers by developing beers with fruity flavors, likely to be better tolerated by younger drinkers.

Considering that excessive alcohol consumption cost the United States $249 billion in 2010—from reduced workplace productivity, increased health-care expenses, and other costs like criminal justice expenses, motor vehicle crash costs, and property damage—amounting to a little over $2 per drink, it might seem we are subsidizing corporate profits. And indeed, in addition to public marketing campaigns, in the United States in 2014 alcoholic beverage companies declared spending $24.7 million on lobbyists and a further $17.1 million on campaign contributions to support particular politicians or parties. Perhaps these cozy relationships are part of the reason that the alcohol beverage industry has been growing at breakneck speed—over a 10 percent increase every five years for the past few decades. If profits are our motive, these strategies are obviously effective, but given the human costs they are morally questionable.

What might we do differently? As a start, we might work to ensure more spaces where not drinking isn't just tolerated but acceptable. In addition to offering more beverage options, we could convey this acceptance by really seeing and hearing each other, putting the "social" back into the drinking. Practicing this, we might notice that at least some of those we meet will be better sated by friendship than by booze.

6

The Downer Class: Tranquilizers

And though she's not really ill
There's a little yellow pill

—Keith Richards and Mick Jagger,
"Mother's Little Helper" (1966)

Mother's Little Helper

Despite the notoriety of illicit drug use in the 1960s and 1970s, addiction to legally prescribed drugs, like those immortalized by the Rolling Stones in their song "Mother's Little Helper," was much more common. The same is true today. The Stones were singing about Miltown, a member of the class of sedative-hypnotics that quickly became a best seller, accounting for a third of all prescriptions written only two years after its introduction in 1955. During the period from 1955 to 1960, billions of Miltown pills were manufactured as people worldwide couldn't seem to get enough pharmacological help. Early on, these drugs were thought to have little addictive risk (incidentally, this was also a halcyon period for tobacco before anyone recognized the link between smoking and cancer). As soon as the patent on one drug was busted, similar ones were in line to take its place. For example, by the 1970s, Valium was the single most prescribed brand of medicine in the United States, used by about one in five women. It was also the cause of more emergency room visits than all illicit drugs combined. Though overdose from Valium is virtually impossible, withdrawal symptoms are anything but banal; combined with tolerance and craving, these drugs are highly addictive. Nonetheless, in 1980, 2.6 billion pills were dispensed, which is almost one hundred doses per person.[1] Since then, minor modifications to the formulations have ensured a steady stream of patentable products, and use of these addictive drugs is higher than ever. In 2013, close to 6 percent of U.S. adults filled more than thirteen million prescriptions for sedative-hypnotics.

The need for this class of drugs was, and is, real. Manic patients including those suffering with bipolar depression or schizophrenia can become stuck in a kind of positive-feedback loop, where delusions increase as sleep decreases. Like an overtired child, some patients find it virtually impossible to rest, while thoughts and behaviors grow more and more problematic. For centuries, involuntary restraint was about the only strategy available to help people calm down, likely adding insult to injury. In the late nineteenth century, opium was introduced as an option and used in cocktails containing multiple plant derivatives—some of which were toxic. The first true sleep medicine was chloral hydrate, perhaps familiar to some as the knockout drops mixed with alcohol to make a Mickey Finn. A series of other compounds, like bromides, were popular for a short time, but all of these drugs had a very narrow therapeutic window. This means that the difference between an effective dose and an overdose is small and in fact gets narrower with repeated use. Until the development of barbiturates, the high toxicity of such drugs simply couldn't be avoided. Their side effects included vomiting, confusion, convulsions, cardiac arrhythmia, and even coma.

Then, in 1864, Adolf von Baeyer (a Nobel recipient for his contributions to organic chemistry) synthesized the first barbiturate in the lab, malonylurea, from urea, a product of urine, and malonic acid, derived from apples. It took about forty years of work, but eventually Baeyer introduced diethyl-barbituric acid,[2] beginning a period of consumer zeal and corporate profits that remains strong to this day. Malonylurea, better known as barbituric acid, was immediately recognized as a way to treat difficult patients, especially those with serious mental illness, but it was also used to treat insomnia and epilepsy and as a surgical anesthetic.

The popularity of barbiturates grew rapidly, and by the 1920s they were virtually the sole treatment for conditions benefiting from sedation. However, in 1960 Valium was introduced, initiating a second wave in this pharmacological revolution. All of these compounds are sedating in that they induce both muscular and psychic relaxation; "hypnotic" refers to their sleep-inducing properties. Because stress, anxiety, and insomnia are such common problems, it makes sense that these drugs have been popular since their introduction. Unfortunately, the problem with all the drugs that have been developed to treat these serious issues thus far is that with regular use they elicit an opponent process, therefore creating the state they were designed to remedy. The insomniac become sleepless. The anxious become wrecks.

Like many people, I liked these drugs well enough and often used them alternately with stimulants—a little up if I had to work or was planning a big night of partying, a little down if I needed to sleep or was just feeling mellow. I figured we'd evolved past natural highs and lows, including conventional stimulants like caffeine, and saw no reason not to titrate my own arousal states, as needed. What I liked most about the downer class was the feeling of distance from my feelings. Somewhere in the middle of my lowest period, my grandfather died and I was invited to the funeral. I loved both my grandfathers a lot; this one seemed to see only good in me, despite the lack of evidence. He worked as a pastry chef for fancy hotels when he emigrated from Switzerland after World War I, and one time he made cookies that spelled out "Happy Birthday, Judy" for a special celebration. He was kind and loving, with bright blue eyes that seemed glad to see me no matter what my condition.

Anyway, I was sorry he died, or at least I thought I should be. I attended his funeral completely numb on quaaludes. At one point, I noticed that everyone in the room looked really sad, and I became worried that my face probably lacked appropriate expression, because I wasn't feeling a thing. In fact, it dawned on me like waking from a dream that I was so wasted I was probably wearing a stupid grin. As I tried to "straighten up" and "act right" (major occupations at the time, along with trying to stay blitzed), I worked to contrive a more fitting countenance, by individually adjusting my features to match those of mourning people. Several years later, in treatment and sober for the first time in years, I finally had an opportunity to mourn and sobbed alone for the better part of two days.

Though hardly recreational in a classic sense, these drugs have tremendous appeal for many of us because feelings can be so darn uncomfortable. How nice just to float along in a perpetual twilight, somehow above the morass of anguish that comes with consciousness. Work was more tolerable, annoyances less irritating, ugliness, pain, and death less unbearable. Like those big comfy pillows they give you when you're pregnant, these drugs produce an illusion of being safe and sound and, for me, numb to any inner experience.

A couple of parallels are worth noting. First is the similarity between the booms in sedative-hypnotic use in the mid- to late twentieth century and opiate use in the early twenty-first. What's in vogue in any era will mirror the social context. Anti-anxiety drugs (benzodiazepines) were especially popular before and during the "liberation movement," as if the stress invoked by raising awareness created a bigger need for checking out (or the other way around: sedatives may help us avoid addressing social or personal injustice). Similarly, the opiate epidemic might reflect a reluctance to deal with suffering—in our own lives, but also in the collective as we slowly come to face our complicity in the world's misery and twenty-four-hour news makes it ever less possible to escape tragedies big and small. Or we might speculate that the decline in the use of tranquilizers, caused mostly by negative press and pressure on doctors to reduce the number of prescriptions written, was related to the rise of alcohol use. It would be no wonder, because these drugs essentially represent alcohol in pill form. My point is, there will always be something available to assuage the need to escape the human experience.

Barbiturates

During the twentieth century, more than twenty-five hundred different barbiturates were synthesized. Of these, about fifty were brought into clinical use (even then, it wasn't easy to make this leap). Their use became very widespread, and they are still the drugs of choice in some serious forms of insomnia and epilepsy.

The name "barbiturate," offered by Baeyer, might have come from his friend Barbara, or been inspired by his celebration of the discovery at a nearby pub frequented by artillery officers who themselves were celebrating the day of their patron, Saint Barbara. At any rate, following Baeyer's laboratory break-through, two German researchers, Josef Freiherr von Mering and Emil Fischer, produced the first barbiturate to come to market. As early as 1882, doctors appreciated the drug's sleep-producing effects, and in 1903 diethyl-barbituric acid was marketed as a sleeping pill under the brand name Veronal. Americans changed the name to barbital in a sleight of hand during World War I to permit manufacture of German products in the United States without having to pay royalties.

Barbital was a wonder drug. The ability to sedate and promote sleep in clinical patients was no small feat. An Italian psychiatrist, Giuseppe Epifanio, was the first to report on this effect in an article published in 1915, though because it was during the war, and in Italian, it wasn't widely appreciated. He wrote to describe the result of giving phenobarbital to a nineteen-year-old girl with resistant manic-depressive psychosis. Not only did she fall into a deep sleep, but she went into an extended remission. Eventually "sleep cures" consisting of prolonged sleep therapy caught on and during the 1920s were the only pharmacological treatment for psychosis. They were also used for autism, delirium tremens, and morphine withdrawal.

Very early on it was recognized that these drugs could help epileptic patients, too. This was discovered accidentally by a doctor who was frustrated that his own sleep was interrupted by epileptic patients having seizures during the night, so he gave them phenobarbital. He was pleasantly surprised to find a dramatic dip in the frequency and intensity of his patients' seizures, many of whom were then able to leave institutions and live relatively normal lives. Phenobarbital is currently the most widely prescribed antiepileptic drug in the world, aptly dubbed "king of the barbiturates."

Many analogs have been synthesized—some that have better efficacy (strength) and shorter action, obviating drowsiness the next day. Soon Amytal (amobarbital), Seconal (secobarbital),

Nembutal (pentobarbital), and Pentothal (thiopental) arrived on the market. In short order, people other than psychiatric or epileptic patients began taking these pills to help them sleep or relax, and a large portion began exploiting some of the non-medicinal benefits—though admittedly it's sometimes hard to make the distinction—and becoming addicted. Despite regulation in 1938 by the U.S. Food and Drug Administration (FDA), these drugs only became more popular. Many also began combining barbiturates with alcohol to increase the effect or took them alternately with stimulants to mitigate drowsiness. More recently, their co-prescription with opiates has been thought to contribute to a surge in lethal overdoses.

By the time the United States entered World War II, Americans were consuming more than a billion barbiturates annually, and as production grew to meet demand, so did addiction and overdose. The ability to relax or sleep "on demand" is broadly appealing but may be especially so for those expected to perform in the public eye. According to her death certificate, Marilyn Monroe died of "acute poisoning by overdose of barbiturates" on August 5, 1962, after taking nearly fifty Nembutals. In 1968 alone, 24.7 million prescriptions for barbiturates were issued in the U.K. Around the same time Jimi Hendrix asphyxiated on his own vomit in London after consuming many times the lethal dose of Vesparax, a combination of two barbiturates plus an antihistamine added to lengthen their duration of action. More recently, Michael Jackson succumbed to a massive dose of Propofol, which his private doctor administered to help him sleep. The very short-acting anesthetic doesn't share the barbiturate structure, but acts in a similar fashion. It's a very good anesthetic because it has a really fast onset and short half-life, but like all these drugs, as well as the rest of Mr. Jackson's pharmacological strategies, doses need to escalate as tolerance develops, making the therapeutic window grow narrower and the risk of accidental overdose grow greater over time.

Speaking of which, both inventors of barbiturates, the chemists Fischer and von Mering, died of overdose after years of dependence. As this liability was increasingly recognized, laws regulating the distribution and sale of barbiturates were enacted. The World Health Organization recommended in the 1950s that withdrawal from the drugs was so problematic that they should only be available by prescription. Nonetheless, in the 1960s there were still hundreds of thousands of addicted individuals, and the United States still produces about thirty pills per person per year, making them, among other things, a convenient choice for committing suicide.

There have been other, intentionally nefarious uses for these drugs. In the mid-1950s, studies in Canada financed by the U.S. Central Intelligence Agency used "psychic driving"—essentially brainwashing by combining propaganda with barbiturates. The media was highly critical of these studies, which either ceased or went underground. In a similar vein, intelligence agencies around the world take advantage of barbiturates' ability to decrease inhibitions. By inhibiting inhibitory control—or turning off the brakes on neural regulation—various members of this class have been tested and sometimes used as "truth serums." Sodium amytal and sodium pentothal were used as coadjutant agents for the exercise of narcoanalysis—psychotherapy conducted during a drugged sleep—which was very widespread around the time of World War II.

The crowning nefarious use of barbiturates is state-administered murder. Thirty-three U.S. states, plus the U.S. military and the federal government, authorize use of the death penalty. The preferred method is by lethal injection, and since 1976, 1,483 executions have been carried out using this method.

A cocktail of three drugs is employed: the barbiturate sodium thiopental is used to induce unconsciousness, another to paralyze muscles, and a third to stop the heartbeat. The U.S. manufacturer of sodium thiopental stopped making the drug after its production moved to Italy and the government there threatened to ban its export unless the company could ensure it was not being used for this purpose. The shortage has somewhat slowed the pace of executions.

Barbiturates are still used for surgical anesthesia, as well as in the treatment of epilepsy, and to help reduce intracranial pressure following traumatic brain injury. However, in the 1960s another class of sedative-hypnotics, also $GABA_A$ agonists, was introduced—benzodiazepines—and these were purported to be much safer and less addictive than their predecessors. Not surprisingly, those claims were overstated. Millions of people are now hooked on benzos, but on the bright side it's not possible to overdose from them alone, so the market is likely to stay strong.

Benzos

The $GABA_A$ receptor is the door that is opened by all sedative-hypnotic drugs. GABA is the most ubiquitous inhibitory neurotransmitter and modulates virtually every brain circuit and all behavior. Hundreds of different drugs act on GABA receptors. Most of these target the $GABA_A$ receptor, which is a complex of five proteins that form a ring around a central pore in the cell membrane that permits chloride ions to pass into the cell. Because chloride is negatively charged, when the receptor is activated by GABA or a copycat drug, the chloride current makes the cell more negative than normal. This reduces the excitability of the neuron and slows down cell-to-cell communication. This makes such drugs an effective treatment for epilepsy. Epilepsy is a disorder characterized by recurrent seizures, due to too much cell-to-cell transmission. Many antiepileptic drugs work by enhancing chloride flow through the GABA$_A$ channel.

GABA$_A$ receptor

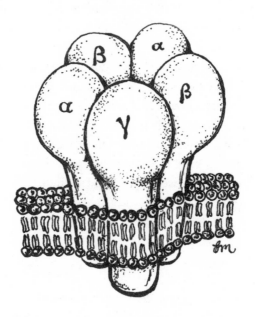

Although all sedative-hypnotics facilitate activity at this receptor, the receptor can vary from person to person. There are nineteen distinct subunits that may assort in the cell membrane to form the receptor complex and well over a thousand possible structures for this single receptor. Each of these structurally distinct receptors has a unique pharmacology—some more or less sensitive to particular drugs, for example.[3] People's individual differences in a drug's rewarding effects, as well as the development of tolerance or dependence, have been associated with structural differences in the GABA$_A$ receptor.[4] For example, whether or not you are able to drink others under the table, or are known as a "lightweight," has been attributed to the particular makeup of subunits. Structural differences may also confer individual variation in pain sensitivity, anxiety, premenstrual or postpartum depression, diagnosis on the autism spectrum, and need for sleep, among others.

So what determines the specific structure of your $GABA_A$ receptor? It depends partly on what we inherit but also on a host of other factors, and this is where things get even more interesting and complicated. Different brain regions and cell types are populated with different receptors, but they also change as a function of our age and developmental period, epigenetic marks related to our ancestors' experiences, and our own experiences—including drug history. The *b process* for all sedative-hypnotics involves modifications to $GABA_A$ receptors so that we can be coherent and upright with the drugs on board (that is, tolerant). But when the drugs are not coursing through our blood and flooding our synapses, the receptors will be grossly understimulated, and we will feel tense and anxious, perhaps to the point of seizing.

The major difference between benzos and barbiturates is that overdose is virtually impossible with benzodiazepines alone and fairly likely with barbiturates. Typically, both drugs act in concert with GABA on its receptor, and so their effects are limited by the presence of GABA in the synapse. But at high doses, barbiturates can mimic GABA and open the chloride channel directly. This allows them to decrease excitation and generally inhibit neurotransmitter release, perhaps to such an extent that the brain activity necessary to life is stopped, and for this reason they are much more toxic. Because of their safety profile, it's relatively simple to get a prescription for a benzodiazepine to treat any anxiety or certain sleep disorders. They may also be used as a muscle relaxant, during alcohol withdrawal, or before surgery to induce relaxation and amnesia. Differences among benzodiazepines are the result of differences in the way they act on the different $GABA_A$ receptor subtypes.

The demand for benzos is higher than ever. Excessive anxiety is estimated to be the sixth leading cause of disability across the globe.[5] Anxiety differs from fear in that the latter is an emotional response to a clear and current danger, as opposed to apprehension about possible future events or unfocused or irrational worry. There are many ways anxiety disorders are expressed, including panic disorder, phobias, obsessive-compulsive disorder, or PTSD (post-traumatic stress disorder). Anxiety disorders are also linked to depression; these are sometimes thought of as two sides of the same underlying issue(s). Anxiety disorders tend to begin early in life and follow a recurrent, intermittent course, exacting costs on life satisfaction, income, education, and relationships. Anxiety is also a major contributor to suicide. On the other hand, at moderate levels anxiety actually improves performance by boosting our energy level and helping us work or focus longer and harder. And anxiety may be an important survival tool because without it we wouldn't be as likely to stay safe. Like many mental disorders, it is thought to reflect an excess of some healthy tendency; neither too little nor too much anxiety is ideal, and we can tell if it is too much when it impedes a person's living to her fullest potential.

Up to a third of the worldwide population suffers from anxiety at some point in their lives, but it is about twice as prevalent in women as in men. In fact, women tend to be two to three times more susceptible to all stress-related disorders, at least partly as a result of neurobiology that is only beginning to be investigated.[6] Drugs used to treat anxiety disorders are called anxiolytics, and these are especially useful for temporary anxiety associated with major life changes like the death of a spouse, divorce, or major surgery. Unfortunately, many people are dependent on benzodiazepines and need them just to function normally. Though they might have begun taking anxiolytics to help them cope with a specific event or stressor, adaptation to these drugs is robust and inevitable, guaranteeing a particularly anxiety-ridden day if one skips a dose. The same is true for those who regularly take any benzodiazepine to help with insomnia. The benefits dwindle over time, at least for patients, if not for pharmaceutical companies. Again, it's a bit of a double bind because, like anxiety, insomnia is a major problem. Around a quarter of adults report insomnia symptoms, and a chronic lack of sleep contributes to increased risk of cardiovascular and metabolic disease (including heart attacks and obesity), cancer, psychiatric illness including substance abuse, and impaired cognition and behavior. In the United States, about two million drivers fall asleep at the wheel every week, and drowsy drivers crash every twenty-five seconds. So obviously a lack of good sleep is problematic. It would be terrific to be able to pop a pill and experience a deep, restful sleep whenever we wanted. Unfortunately, unless this is a rare practice, the opponent process makes it impossible. On the first night, the drug does work like a charm, quickly and effectively transporting one to the land of nod. But like all drugs that produce their effects by altering activity of the brain, the honeymoon period doesn't last long.

Downregulation of $GABA_A$ receptor sensitivity is produced by decreasing the number of receptors on the cell surface as well as changes in the subunit constituency, and both of these contribute to tolerance.[7] Where half a milligram used to do the trick, you now need two. But worse than this is the fact that it becomes harder and harder to get anything like a decent night's sleep without the drug. You could try switching prescriptions, but this too will be futile. Any regular user can prove it so by skipping a night (however, no cheating with the liquid form, alcohol!). Lying in bed desperate for rest, the chronic user of benzodiazepines is likely to experience the phenomenon of craving as strongly as any other addict.

Given all this, it might be surprising to know that prescriptions for benzodiazepines are on the rise. This is due partly to our proclivity for seeking pharmacological solutions to our problems and partly to corporate eagerness to respond to, even nurture, that tendency. A recent report found that between 1996 and 2013 the number of benzodiazepine prescriptions increased 67 percent, and the total quantity of benzodiazepines filled by pharmacies more than tripled during the same period due to the fact that more people are taking more pills.[8] Besides addiction, the risks associated with this pattern include falls and other accidents, such as vehicle crashes and overdose (when combined with other drugs).

The drug historian Nicolas Rasmussen points out that "the history of tranquilizers is an endless cycle of 'product innovation,' to put it neutrally, with each one pretending to have no side effects and be non-addictive. Then, when these properties are discovered, the drug companies just [promote a] new one."[9] From a neuroscience perspective, the robust and unavoidable *b process* universally elicited by any $GABA_A$ agonist makes these drugs unsuitable for regular use.

It might be a good time to ask, given our long and ardent relationship with this class of drugs despite their substantial liabilities, whether there is a better way to help those suffering with insomnia or anxiety. Or even to wonder how these conditions are so common as to be statistically normal—indeed they afflict at least one in three adults in the United States—yet still are considered abnormal behaviors. One possibility is that some people are more sensitive, or more exposed, than others to environmental factors that contribute to these conditions. For example, a growing scientific consensus suggests that overexposure to light such as that emanating from our beloved screens disrupts circadian rhythms to adversely affect a range of health outcomes including mood and sleep.[10] Twenty years into a second century of abuse of this class of mainly prescription drugs, it might be time to look for alternative ways of coping—especially ones that don't make the problem worse.

7

Pick-Me-Ups: Stimulants

There's no happy ending to cocaine.
You either die, you go to jail, or else you
run out.

—Sam Kinison (1953–1992)

Universal

As a class of drugs that increase movement, stimulants are the most popular mind-altering drugs worldwide and in many ways have been the low-hanging fruit of the addictive drug family. Users have been enjoying natural stimulants from amphetamine-producing plants such as *Catha edulis* (khat) and *Ephedra sinica* (ma huang) for at least several thousand years. In contrast to that of sedative-hypnotics, a group of drugs that share both action and effects, stimulant classification is based solely on effect. The stimulant class is large and diverse and could easily be topic enough for an entire book, but this chapter will focus on caffeine, nicotine, cocaine, the amphetamines, and 3,4-methylenedioxymethamphetamine, or MDMA. The last three of these—coke, amphetamines, and ecstasy—are somewhat low-hanging fruit for researchers, too, because they all work very precisely through the same general mechanism to alter neural activity.

Stimulants increase general arousal and alertness, which is to say that most of us have an easier time focusing and staying alert with these drugs on board. The fact that everyone likes to be stimulated accounts for some of their wide use, but it also has to do with the fact that caffeine and nicotine are both legal and largely unregulated. In addition, there are not many contexts in which being alert and active is contraindicated. Drugs that produce effects like sleep, hallucinations, or dissociation, on the other hand, obviously garner less social acceptance.

The stimulants methylphenidate (Ritalin) and amphetamine (Adderall) have been effectively used to treat attention deficit hyperactivity disorder (ADHD) for almost sixty years. ADHD diagnoses are common: in the United States, about 12 percent of children over age four have a diagnosis for an attention deficit disorder, and most of these, about four million, are treated with stimulants each day.[1] The difference between those with ADHD diagnoses and those without is quantitative: for those with the disorder, drug treatment brings their cognition within normal range. Nonetheless, the high rates of use of these drugs in clinical populations, as well as by many in the normal range looking for enhancement rather than treatment, have led to concerns about possible long-term effects, and especially to the fear that the treatment may increase the risk for subsequently developing addiction. Given what we know about adaptation, it seems especially plausible because these drugs increase dopamine levels throughout the brain, including in the nucleus accumbens. In general, though, the research suggests that when these drugs are used as prescribed for ADHD, chronic exposure to them does not have lasting effects on behavior or cognition.[2]

Most abused drugs interact in multiple neural pathways, and with many of these drugs, people don't find the balance of effects to be a net positive. Alcohol, THC, and even opiates are notorious for producing variable effects; some of us like them all, but many people have strong preferences for one or another. This is generally not the case with the classic stimulants: cocaine and the amphetamines. Multiple studies have shown that when these substances are administered in a controlled laboratory setting, virtually everybody enjoys their effects. (The primary difference between the two is that the amphetamine high lasts much longer.)

That enjoyment doesn't survive repeated use. Cocaine and amphetamine are especially noteworthy for their unique patterns of adaptation to long-term use. As always with addictive drugs, tolerance spoils the fun, in this case as dopamine levels dip below normal levels, and often stay depleted after a binge. However, other drug effects, including those associated with movement and cognition, tend to get more robust rather than less so with repeated exposures, a phenomenon called sensitization. Sensitization among stimulant users is thought to account for bizarre behavioral and cognitive changes that often develop over time, such as stereotypy. Stereotypy is evident as highly dosed or sensitized individuals engage in purposeless, repetitive movement. There can be other causes of stereotypical behavior besides drugs, but it is common enough among speed users to have its own slang: users often refer to stereotypies as punding or tweaking, as they mindlessly sort, clean, or dis- and reassemble objects, for example. Other long-term effects are even more alarming. Drugs classified as stimulants are sympathomimetics; that is, they stimulate the sympathetic branch of the autonomic nervous system, which can interfere with sleep and put strain on the cardiovascular system. In some cases, psychiatric conditions may emerge in chronic users, such as stimulant psychosis, which may result from sensitization of cognitive arousal to the point of paranoia and hallucinations. This usually, but not always, resolves with abstinence.

Another quirk of stimulant use is that over repeated exposures there is often a growing aversion to the drug, so that what initially presented as pure pleasure becomes an ambivalent mix of wanting and not wanting, measured in the lab by compulsive approach behavior as well as avoidant behavior. The more exposure to the drug one has, the larger the conflict grows. This pattern of approach-avoidance tends not to be seen with other drugs like alcohol or opiates and has a fascinating animal model.[3] Rats will readily learn to run up an alley for a cocaine infusion. In one study, they have this opportunity once a day for fourteen consecutive days, but instead of going faster each day, as they would with other drugs such as heroin, they begin quickly and just before reaching the infusion source are apt to turn and run the other way. They usually go back and forth several times—"Yes! I want it" / "No! I don't"—suggesting to researchers what every addict already appreciates: that cocaine addiction is a mix of positive and negative motivational states and that the negative consequences sensitize. Some have hypothesized that this quirky and unfortunate adaptation may account for the association between cocaine use and anxiety disorders, which emerge with frequent use and grow worse as the addiction progresses. To make the point that the "Yes" virtually always wins, giving people unlimited access to cocaine often results in uncontrolled binges and eventually death. Neither is the case with opiates or alcohol. Although overdoses to those drugs can occur, they don't happen from refusing to stop, maybe in part because with enough of those drugs, dopers and alcoholics at least fall asleep.

Caffeine

Caffeine is the most popular psychoactive drug in the world, although there is some debate about whether or not it is addictive. Though regular use may result in a modicum of tolerance and will likely cause dependence (that is, withdrawal upon abstinence) and craving, the drug is not considered harmful, thus skipping one of the core criterion for addiction. In fact, there are several documented benefits to regular caffeine use including improvements in mood, memory, alertness, and physical and cognitive performance. It also seems to reduce the risk of developing Parkinson's disease and type 2 diabetes. This is all good news, especially because, unlike many other psychoactive substances, it is legal and unregulated nearly everywhere.

The pharmacological effects of caffeine are similar to those of other members of its subclass, the methylxanthines, which are also found in various teas and chocolates. Methylxanthines are made by a number of plants native to South America and East Asia. Effects of caffeine and other methylxanthines include mild CNS stimulation and wakefulness, an increase in the ability to sustain concentration, and quicker reaction times. The most well-known source of caffeine is the *Coffea* plant, and it's actually the seeds, not the beans, that are roasted and ground to satisfy the large and growing demand. The drug is very safe—one would need to quickly consume about a hundred cups to reach a lethal dose—and desired effects begin a few minutes after consuming the beverage and peak about an hour later. The half-life is fairly long, about four to nine hours, with the large range attributed mostly to genetic differences influencing metabolism. Again, the half-life refers to the amount of time it takes to get rid of (usually metabolize) 50 percent of the drug, so it's worth remembering this if you have problems sleeping but like to spend time in the café.

On the other hand, the drug is widely appreciated for its ability to delay or prevent sleep and to improve performance of simple tasks during times of significant sleep deprivation. Therefore, shift workers who use caffeine make fewer mistakes than those who don't. It also improves athletic performance and endurance, benefiting athletes as well as those of us just trying to make use of the gym. In moderate doses, caffeine may elevate mood and reduce symptoms of depression.

Though there aren't many drawbacks to the drug, it does increase the risk of miscarrying and may cause a rise in blood pressure. Moreover, even when it is taken at moderate doses some people have mild unpleasant symptoms such as anxiety, jitteriness, insomnia, and taking longer to fall asleep. At very high doses (like five NoDoz tablets, or about fifteen cups of coffee), people experience restlessness, irritability possibly progressing to delirium, vomiting, increased respiration, and perhaps convulsions. In addition to acting on the brain, caffeine affects the functioning of the cardiovascular, respiratory, and renal systems. Caffeine dependence can involve withdrawal symptoms such as fatigue, headache, irritability, depressed mood, inability to concentrate, and drowsiness. About half the people who drink it regularly will experience headaches if they suddenly withdraw.

The mechanism by which caffeine produces its effects is not completely understood, but we do know that it doesn't act like cocaine, amphetamine, or MDMA to directly enhance the transmission of dopamine, norepinephrine, and/or serotonin. Instead, caffeine is an antagonist at adenosine receptors (just as Narcan is an antagonist at opiate receptors). Adenosine may be familiar in its role in adenosine triphosphate, or ATP, a primary source of energy. But adenosine also serves as a neurotransmitter and is thought to build up over the day, accumulating in synapses where it binds to its receptors, precipitating a state of drowsiness. When caffeine is on board, adenosine signaling is blocked and as a result temporarily prevents or relieves drowsiness and maintains or restores alertness.

Unless I count chocolate or hot sauce, caffeine is the only

substance left me to manipulate my psychological states. I wish I could say I could take it or leave it, but that is anything but the truth. My home is filled with coffee paraphernalia including a special grinder that I sometimes take along in my suitcase, a special filter and water preparatory machine, and even particular cups. My "bottom" occurred on a camping trip in the desert. Though I had plenty of water, I didn't anticipate my stove breaking. I was fine eating cold refried beans and oats, but what was I going to do without coffee? It wasn't pretty: on the second morning after going cold turkey, I decided to simply eat the ground beans and choked down a heaping spoonful. They weren't delicious, and my gritty smile wasn't beautiful, but I began to feel better within about fifteen minutes. Later it bothered me: Why get clean and free from other drugs but keep this habit? So I made myself give it up, which lasted for a while, until I traveled to Guatemala, where they grow and serve the most delicious coffee, with hot milk. I told myself I was just "doing as the locals do" and then decided to buy three pounds to take home, where I vowed to make them last a few months. Instead, I went straight back to my fiendish ways and then had to find a new supplier because my tastes had progressed.

Nicotine

According to the World Health Organization, over 1.1 *billion* people smoke tobacco, and more than 7 million die each year from their addiction. Like every addict who dies gradually, it isn't because they over-enjoyed a good thing. Instead, the misery imposed by an adapted brain makes quitting seem worse than dying. Though I'm also a former smoker and can therefore be self-righteous, I don't think nicotine is worth dying for.

On average, tobacco users lose fifteen years of life. Today,

5.7 percent of total health expenditures are spent treating smoking-related illnesses, and 12 percent of all adult deaths worldwide result from this habit. In fact, the total annual cost of smoking is almost 2 percent of global gross domestic product, which is also about 40 percent of what all the world's governments spent on education.[4] In total, nicotine addiction burdens the global economy with more than $1.4 trillion in health care and lost productivity each year.

The good news is that with few exceptions (for example, the eastern Mediterranean and African countries) smoking rates are decreasing. This decline is fastest in countries where people experience high self-efficacy, but is holding steady or even increasing in those places where an individual's efforts are unlikely to benefit their situation. (Self-efficacy is higher in places where it's possible to make a living wage, contribute to a family or community, and look forward to the future.) Fewer people in the United States are smoking, though it still remains the number one preventable cause of sickness and mortality in this country. In 2013 about 21 percent of Americans over eleven were current cigarette smokers, and in 2016 just shy of 20 percent still smoked. The positive trend may reflect switching to e-cigarettes or marijuana. Either of these is likely to be less harmful to physical health, primarily because the vehicle for nicotine—as well as much of the taste and smell qualities in smoked tobacco—is tar, which is well known to be carcinogenic. We don't really know about the long-term effects of e-cigarettes, and the drawbacks of habitual marijuana use are likely to be more emotional and cognitive than physical, at least relative to cigarettes. Though teen smoking is declining most rapidly, with over a 7 percent drop from 2002 to 2013, during that period more than twice as many twelfth graders had smoked weed as tobacco in the previous month (22.5 percent versus 10.5 percent), reflecting a change of substance perhaps more than a change of habit. Nonetheless, about half the world's children are regularly exposed to secondhand smoke, which has been definitively linked to a range of health hazards. While on the topic of children, about 1.3 million are exploited through tobacco farming, which further exposes them to pesticides, rife on tobacco fields. The drug is a beast.

Tobacco is native to the Americas and was first domesticated more than five thousand years ago in South America. Cigarette smoking took off in Europe in the mid-nineteenth century, and especially after the invention of automated rollers, which made cigarettes much faster to produce: a skilled worker could make up to three thousand butts a day, but the machine could make at least twice that every *minute*. Nicotine is vaporized by high temperatures at the burning tip of a cigarette and enters the lungs on tiny particles of tar, or it is delivered in vaporized form in electronic cigarettes. Once in the lungs, it is readily absorbed into the bloodstream and distributed to the brain in about seven seconds. (A pack a day smoker takes in over two hundred separate hits of nicotine a day.) It is believed nicotine is highly addictive in part because of its rapid onset of action. A cigarette contains between six and eleven milligrams of nicotine, though much less than this actually reaches the bloodstream of a smoker because most of the drug is metabolized to cotinine in the liver by a specific enzyme called cytochrome P450 2A6 (CYP2A6) and excreted in the urine. Some people have a mutation in the gene that makes CYP2A6 that slows down nicotine metabolism. Because the drug hangs around longer, these people are less likely to become smokers, but if they do, they smoke fewer cigarettes than people who have normal levels of this enzyme.

This may seem counterintuitive—wouldn't more nicotine in the system promote addiction rather than retard it? As with all drug addictions, the target concentration is an ideal window between withdrawal and toxicity. Nicotine is metabolized fairly quickly, and a smoker has to regularly dose to avoid withdrawal, but there is such a thing as too much nicotine. When I smoked, the day was broken up into between-cigarette-intervals rather than minutes or hours (though of course there was a high correlation between these things). However, I suspect I have the mutation in CYP2A6, because if I smoked too much, I would feel a little queasy and clammy. I remember (after I'd quit) taking a road trip with a good friend who definitely had the efficient variant, as well as a mean dependence. We were driving through gorgeous southwest canyon country, but after a while all I could focus on was the countdown to her next reach. She was more reliable than Big Ben.

Most regular smokers consume two to three cigarettes an hour; I was closer to two, while my friend lit up every fourteen minutes (plus or minus a few seconds). Though either pattern leads to ever-increasing levels of nicotine across the day (because each butt takes about two hours to metabolize), the drug doesn't cause greater and greater effects due to the rapid development of tolerance. Though some diehards wake for a bump in the middle of the night to keep withdrawal at bay, most wait to light up after they get up and receive a payoff for their patience. The dynamic adaptations that lead to tolerance within such a short time are mirrored on the other end as tolerance partially decreases during even a few hours of withdrawal, so the first few puffs are the best of the day. The bigger lesson here is the temporal symmetry: tolerance that develops rapidly tends to reverse quickly too, while changes that take longer to accrue tend to persist.

Nicotine is classified as a stimulant, even though every regular smoker knows it helps them to relax and deal with stress.

This is related to rapid tolerance. Nicotine works first to stimulate acetylcholine receptors, but they quickly respond by becoming insensitive, leading to the bidirectional effects of the drug. There are two major types of acetylcholine receptors, and nicotine interacts with only one: aptly named the nicotinic acetylcholine receptor, or nAChR. A cousin of the $GABA_A$ receptor, nAChRs are also made of five subunits that surround a central pore. This receptor permits the flow of sodium, rather than chloride, and because sodium ions carry a positive charge, nAChRs are excitatory. Nicotine activates these receptors by substituting for acetylcholine and thereby increasing neuronal activity. Also reminiscent of the $GABA_A$ receptor, much of the structural and functional diversity of nAChRs arises from the many possible subunit combinations; in this case, there are sixteen different subunits. These combine to form different nAChR subtypes, which have different patterns of expression throughout the brain as well as diverse functional properties and unique pharmacological characteristics. Because acetylcholine signaling is also pervasive, and nAChR expression is extremely broad, practically every area of the brain is affected by nicotine. However, unlike the $GABA_A$ receptor that can be either closed or open, the nAChR has three states: closed, open, and desensitized. The open state is responsible for the stimulant properties of the drug, while the desensitized state produces a cigarette's calming effects. The rate at which the receptor moves through these states and its ability to conduct a positive current depend on the subunit composition. And at least one functional variant modifies the risk for becoming a chronic smoker. Though much of this is still being worked out, it seems clear that genetic variation in the subunit(s) structure of the nAChR accounts for a substantial amount of the risk for nicotine dependence.[5] In the nucleus accumbens, receptors with the a6 subunit seem to be especially involved in maintaining prolonged activation of dopamine neurons and thus encourage addiction.

Like other addictive substances, nicotine initiates addiction by stimulating mesolimbic dopamine pathways, but cigarette smoking affects multiple processes including thinking and attention, learning and memory, emotion, arousal, and motivation because of the distribution of nAChRs in circuits that contribute to all these behaviors. Some of these effects have led to the idea that a nicotine patch might be used to treat cognitive decline in the elderly—the drug can improve some aspects of attention and memory—but the unlikelihood of being able to take anything long term without incurring compensatory adaptations, or substantial side effects, has so far kept these out of the clinic.

It is notoriously hard to quit smoking, a combination of habits being hard to change and nicotine's particular form of withdrawal. After chronic exposure, withdrawal produces a profound syndrome of craving characterized by irritability, anxiety, attention deficits, trouble sleeping, and increased appetite. The reason for this, of course, is the *b process,* which in smokers is largely accounted for by an upregulation of nAChRs. Usually we think that a drug that acts as an agonist by stimulating receptors as nicotine does would produce a downregulation. Why should activating a receptor cause it to become more sensitive and more numerous? Though at first it may seem contrary, recall that nicotine's long-lasting presence results mostly in nAChR desensitization, and the homeostatic response to desensitized receptors is upregulation. So what is the effect of all those extra-sensitive nicotinic receptors? Because nAChRs affect the release of virtually every major transmitter, neuroadaptations from chronic exposure lead to widespread and general alterations in neurotransmission throughout the brain.[6]

Many neurotransmitters that are regulated by acetylcholine transmission such as glutamate, GABA, dopamine, and opioids have their activity altered by the changes in acetylcholine signaling, and all of this adjustment combines to produce the experience of dependence. When the drug is withdrawn these adaptive changes are no longer needed and lead to physical and emotional symptoms of withdrawal within a few hours.

A final note about this popular drug concerns its frequent dance partner: alcohol. Many people notice that drinking makes them want to smoke, or vice versa, and wonder why this is. There are several hypotheses, each of which may explain part of the relationship. For one, any drug that stimulates dopamine greases the rails for another. Because they are both addictive, they can also serve as reminders of addiction, and especially when smoking was okay in bars, the contextual cues were largely overlapping. Also, the arousing effects of nicotine may counteract the sedative effects of alcohol, reflecting the familiar pattern of users counterbalancing uppers and downers. One more hypothesis suggests that smokers can drink more, perhaps because nicotine stimulates digestion and this might decrease alcohol absorption from the gut. So, until further study, we're not sure whether, overall, the two drugs enhance or counteract each other's effects.

Coke

Giving up drugs was really difficult. I was miserable when I quit smoking, especially for the first few days, and then I craved a cigarette every time I was stressed, and decades later I still occasionally wish for the pleasure and relaxation that come with a smoke. I missed drinking every day for fourteen months, white-knuckling my way through constant longing while substituting copious amounts of Ben and Jerry's. Weed was even worse, as I might have mentioned. My relationship with cocaine was more like leaving a mean, unfaithful lover. Pangs of desperate regret mixed with a growing sense of relief. It was like most users of coke and meth in that my compulsion was repulsive even to me, yet I'd have kept on, grinding my jaw tighter, had it not been for Steve's brief epiphany that probably saved my life. He was the friend who noted with unexpected insight that there wasn't enough cocaine in the world to satisfy our desire, and somehow—I honestly have no idea how—steered us both away from injecting over the ensuing several months that it took me to get to treatment.

My love-hate relationship is typical and is thought to reflect the opponent process.[7] At first the drug produces a thrilling rush of euphoria, but this is quickly followed by anxiety, depression, and craving for more drug. Cocaine is like the sole porn shop in a down-and-out town. You hate yourself for going but end up visiting over and over. While using, especially in a binge, I felt as if I were flooring the gas pedal, headed for a granite wall, unable or unwilling to stop, or even to care. It was the short course to self-loathing, and with every bag my soul grew more and more hollow. Cocaine is the drug I miss the least.

The mechanism of cocaine's action is so straightforward compared with most other drugs it seems impossibly simple. On the other hand, the specificity of its action on the nervous system is what makes its effects so effective. Of all the drugs discussed so far, this one has the fewest "side effects," and I often wonder whether the drug's efficiency accounted for my early bottom. What goes up, must come down, as we've seen, and with coke the slope is equally steep in both directions. I have a feeling I'd have gone on longer if my primary relationship had been with alcohol, or even opiates. Despite its action being specific and well known, there are no FDA-approved pharmacotherapies for cocaine addiction.

Cocaine, the amphetamines (including methamphetamine), and ecstasy all have a very similar mechanism of action. Unlike many of the drugs we've discussed, including caffeine and nicotine, but also THC, opiates, and sedative-hypnotics, their primary action—that is, the one responsible for their desired effects—does not involve interacting with a receptor. Instead, they interfere with the recycling mechanism for monoamine neurotransmitters. Though the name monoamine might be new, most people are familiar with the members of this group of neurotransmitters: dopamine, norepinephrine, epinephrine (or adrenaline), serotonin, and melatonin, chemicals that play major roles in mood and sleep.

Monoamines and transporter substrates

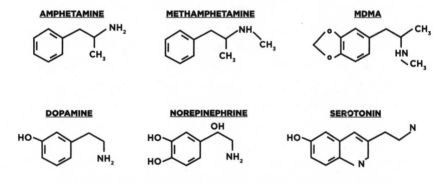

Coke, speed, and E all act by blocking transporters. Transporters, like receptors, are proteins embedded in the neural cell membrane, but unlike receptors the function of transporters is to transport (or recycle) released neurotransmitter back into the presynaptic neuron, where it can be repackaged and reused. Transporters are one of the two main ways that synaptic transmission is discontinued; the other is through enzymatic degradation.

Without transporters or enzymes to break apart neurotransmitters, synaptic transmission would persist much longer than it does, and therefore the signal would be quite different. When one of these drugs occupies a spot on a transporter, it prevents the monoamines from utilizing their reuptake mechanism and prolongs their effects. In the case of dopamine, for example, indication of something newsworthy would be more like a home alarm than a pop-up notification.

A monoamine synapse

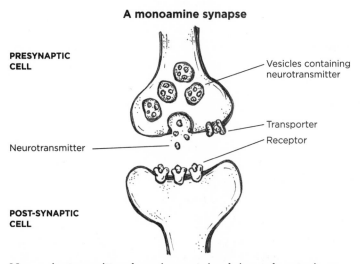

Monoamine transmitters dopamine, norepinephrine, and serotonin are released from vesicles into the synaptic gap and interact with receptors to produce their effects. They may be degraded by enzymes or transported back into the presynaptic cell, for reuse. Cocaine, amphetamines, and MDMA (ecstasy) block transporters, thus prolonging transmitter effects. Amphetamines and MDMA can also be transported into cells by the recycling mechanism, perhaps accounting for their potent neurotoxicity.

That's it. Thousands of people have lost their families, jobs, homes, and lives because the ability of cocaine to extend dopamine's presence in the synapse seemed worth giving up relatively unimportant stimuli like relationships, a livelihood, and teeth. The half-life is very short (usually less than an hour), and though pharmacologists say the subjective effects last about thirty minutes, in my experience it was more like three, barely enough time to prepare the next bump.

What's more, the abuse of cocaine, which may be snorted, swallowed, smoked, or shot, will, depending on the route of administration, increase risk of cardiorespiratory disease, seizures, stroke, and infection; it may also damage nasal cartilage and increase the risk of autoimmune disorders. Snorting gets a relatively sluggish response (though it is still effective, as is oral consumption), but by either inhalation or injection the drug blocks reuptake of monoamines within seconds. IV use is also associated with the transmission of other diseases such as hepatitis C and HIV/AIDS. Abuse of methamphetamine produces similar effects as well as marked degeneration of dopaminergic neurons, resulting in an increased risk for Parkinson's disease.

All abused drugs are compelling, at least to some people under some circumstances, but coke is probably the most universally enjoyable substance yet discovered. At the peak of my cocaine use, I lived in Parkland, Florida, sharing a house with several other people like me for the better part of a year. I think I actually had only two other official roommates, though it was hard to tell: Laurie, whose name was on the lease and didn't like to buy but stayed well supplied by renting rooms to people like me; and Tommy, a better housemate from Laurie's perspective than I was. Tommy was from a long line of dealers. As I remember it, his grandmother was doing hard time, and at least one of his parents was dead (he wasn't certain about the other). I'm sure the area is thoroughly tamed by now, but in the mid-1980s, except for the lack of elevation, it felt like an Andean outpost. Riding a bicycle one day, I was stopped by a guy in military garb holding a machine gun who let me know the road was closed. I think I briefly objected because it was a public road, but for once even I could tell it would be stupid to argue. The whole place was totally unpredictable, and at times I saw enough helicopter traffic to make it seem like a regional hospital. I ended up there because, one night after my waitressing shift at a chain restaurant, I arrived home in Delray, my previous abode, to find my stuff packed and sitting in the driveway. I didn't know or couldn't remember what I had done to warrant such treatment, but my roommates—somewhat prudish and boring, I thought— were allied in their position, meeting me with crossed arms and impassive faces. That I was easily able to find the room in Parkland speaks to the implicit kinship among users; the further away from social norms I traveled, the easier it was to connect with my kind, just as water flows to the lowest point.

I came home one night to find Tommy hiding behind a palm tree (we were all pretty skinny) with an AK-47. His eyes looked like CDs—huge, flat, and totally crazy. I could tell he'd been up for a while, not only by the way he looked, but because he was well into a paranoid delusion about people trying to steal his dogs. He had two beautiful Rottweilers, Roxy and Bear, that he certainly didn't deserve. He was sure there were people lurking around the property and his gun was cocked and loaded, but my brain turned instead to the problem of how much drug remained and how I was going to get it. Luckily, he hadn't used it all. Unluckily, someone—probably pissed over a deal—shot the dogs about a week later.

Meth

Methamphetamine abuse is a significant problem worldwide. Though rates in the United States have been stable with about a million chronic users, the market is growing quickly in East and Southeast Asia.[8] Meth is a Schedule II drug and may be prescribed for ADHD, extreme obesity, and narcolepsy, but amphetamine is more often the choice of physicians because it is less reinforcing than methamphetamine (the addition of a methyl group increases absorption and distribution). Either of these drugs can be neurotoxic when taken at high doses, and there is no treatment for this brain damage. Adderall, a popular choice for ADHD, is a form of amphetamine, often delivered in a slow-release formulation.

The United Nations Office on Drugs and Crime indicates that meth is one of the most popular synthetic drugs worldwide, with at least thirty-seven million users—about twice the number of either cocaine or heroin (with about seventeen million users each). The first broad use of methamphetamine was as an over-the-counter decongestant and bronchodilator, and right from the start some clever users figured out how to remove the drug-soaked cotton plug at the bottom of the inhaler to quickly deliver high doses. The next big surge in use, also before the abuse potential was widely recognized, occurred during World War II, when all three superpowers (Japan, Germany, and the United States) might have been so as a result of loading their troops with "uppers." After the war, veterans from these countries continued to use the drug, which wasn't much regulated for the next couple of decades. Once legitimate synthesis and distribution slowed in the 1960s, however, these tasks were taken over by clandestine labs. By 1990, methamphetamine was more popular than cocaine and went to the top of the DEA's war on drugs list. As most are aware, regulation, legislation, and prosecution haven't made much of a dent, and kitchen-based meth labs are more or less able to keep up with demand. My friend Steve had more than ten times the lethal dose of methamphetamine in his blood when he died.

The half-life of methamphetamine is about ten hours (ten times that of cocaine), but amphetamine's half-life varies widely—anywhere from seven to thirty hours, depending on the pH of the user's urine. Behavioral effects don't typically last that long, because all this overstimulation leads to acute tolerance as synapses get depleted of monoamines. The effects from acute low to moderate doses include euphoria, "rush," wakefulness, antifatigue, increased confidence, hyperactivity, and loss of appetite. Higher doses also cause talkativeness, aggressiveness, restlessness, and stereotypy. Very high doses (such as those experienced during a binge) may cause agitation, confusion, anxiety, irritability, dysphoria, violent behavior, impaired psychomotor and cognitive skills, hallucinations, stereotypy, paranoia, or skin crawling. During the end of a binge, users experience extreme dysphoria and anxiety as well as a sense of emptiness. The acute withdrawal phase tends to improve over the next few days—especially with sleep and food—and things often return to the status quo. In contrast to most other drugs, where there is more or less a linear relationship between time since last using and the experience of craving, with coke and meth craving seems to build over time, and most users relapse within a few weeks.

Several years after getting clean, I had a friend who also struggled with a stimulant addiction. She was a beautiful woman, and talented, whose greatest joy was being with her daughter. We'd usually talk toward the end of her binge, when her desolation was so deep it seemed to seep through the cellular waves. She'd swear off the drug, regretting that she'd spent the money she needed to buy her daughter a birthday present, further compromised her health, or put her job at risk. She'd even go so far as to block the dealer's number. Days would pass as she'd begin to get her life together; smart and resourceful, she was amazingly capable of righting the boat during these many periods.

But inevitably—most often on a biweekly basis that coincided with a paycheck, but not always, sometimes calling but sometimes not—she'd eventually succumb to her addiction. From the outside, it looked like someone picking up speed (pun intended) while swimming hard toward a waterfall. She'd describe the imminent fall, full of sadness and anxiety, as if watching someone she formerly loved lose the battle against a bacterial infection. Sometimes she'd report, just before going off-line, "I'm going to relapse, so I might as well get it over with," as she'd wave good-bye for her several-day trip over the chute, unblocking the dealer who seemed always prepared to take full advantage of the cheerless routine. Her life was a seesaw of remorse and compulsion, pivoting on a fulcrum of despair.

This sounds very much like the pattern of approach-avoidance seen in animal studies discussed at the beginning of the chapter. My beautiful friend's addiction quickly devolved into tolerance to meth's euphoric effects, while sensitization to cognitive stress systems made her using feel like torture, the way a hungry lab rat must feel about having to endure a shock to get food.

Ecstasy

MDMA is sometimes classified as a stimulant and sometimes as a hallucinogen; in fact, it's a little bit of both. Because I never had the opportunity to try this drug, I won't pretend to be an expert on its subjective effects, but in terms of chemical structure and mechanism of action it fits more squarely with the stimulants. Amphetamine, methamphetamine, and MDMA all acutely interact with monoamine transporters to block reuptake and cause release of dopamine, norepinephrine, and serotonin from nerve terminals, although MDMA has a relatively greater effect on the serotonin system. Pure MDMA does share some pharmacological properties with mescaline, one of the classic psychedelic drugs that will be discussed in the next chapter. This similarity, both structurally and functionally, is hoped by some to indicate potential therapeutic benefits of the drug, which was recently approved for its first clinical trial in the United States. Ecstasy is not at all similar to LSD or psilocybin, though, and like that of other stimulants its ability to block reuptake of monoamines is what leads to enhanced energy, endurance, sociability, and sexual arousal, justifying its reputation as a perfect party drug.

The major distinction from amphetamine and methamphetamine is the methylenedioxy ($-O-CH_2-O-$) group, which is what makes it resemble mescaline. Like amphetamine, however, MDA and MDMA are synthetic; amphetamine was developed in 1885, MDA in 1910, and MDMA just a couple of years later. In 1985, MDA and MDMA were placed in Schedule I in the United States, and they are similarly classified in Canada (Schedule III) and the U.K. (Class A). The DEA and the FDA work together to determine which substances belong in which schedules, ranging from I to V depending on the drug's acceptable medical use and the drug's abuse or dependency potential. Schedule I drugs are considered to have the highest potential for abuse and dependence and Schedule V the least. But don't let the government's involvement suggest careful supervision of what is for sale. Chemical-grade MDMA often differs substantially from the ecstasy that is bought and sold in the public domain. Because you're more likely than not to buy pills that are adulterated with other stimulants or psychoactives, recreational users often participate in pharmacological roulette.

MDMA is usually taken by mouth or snorted; by mouth it reaches peak concentration in the blood after about two hours and has a fairly long half-life of about eight hours. (As a rule of thumb, it takes about five half-lives to get rid of about 95 percent of *any* drug, so this one hangs around for a couple of days.) Within an hour of MDMA administration, there is a whopping increase in serotonin and other monoamines, followed by a reduction below baseline that develops over days as the drug is slowly metabolized. As a result, people frequently experience aftereffects like lethargy, depression, and memory or concentration problems a few days after "rolling."

But for many, the acute effects make this short-term dip well worth a little low. The drug greatly enhances a sense of well-being and produces extroversion and feelings of happiness and closeness to others, due in part to the fact that it impairs recognition of negative emotions, including sadness, anger, and fear. Affective neuroscience (the study of the brain's role in moods and feelings) has demonstrated quite clearly that we can't feel what we can't recognize, so this pro-social bias seems perfectly engineered and helps explain why ecstasy is called the love drug and has been adopted for use by marriage counselors. In terms of unpleasant acute effects, the drug can cause overheating, teeth grinding, muscle stiffness, lack of appetite, and restless legs—none of which are especially contraindicated on a dance floor.

At concerts I frequent, E is a popular choice, and I imagine it enhances the sensory experience of the lights and guitar riffs as well as the general sense of camaraderie in the pit. As a bystander to this form of enhancement, I certainly appreciate the random hugs and loving vibes of molly users more than the loud sloppiness of the drunks or even the nearly comatose "peacefulness" of the weed heads. In fact, sometimes I think that if it wasn't for the ecstasy users, the only people left dancing during the encore would be the sober ones (and there's more than you might think!). So as far as the acute experience goes, it seems pretty good all around.

But, alas, the more you take any drug, the larger the *b process* grows, and the opponent/dark side of this drug is truly awful. Many regular users look to be headed for a lifetime of depression and anxiety. Research in rats and primates indicates that moderate to high doses of MDMA damage nerve terminals, perhaps permanently. For example, primates given ecstasy twice a day for four days (eight total doses) show reductions in the number of serotonergic neurons *seven years later.*

MDMA neurotoxicity

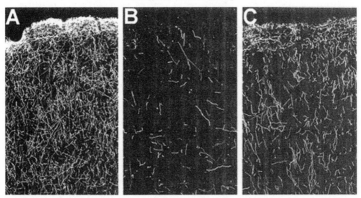

Staining for serotonin neurons in the cortex from a monkey treated with saline (A), two weeks after an MDMA exposure of 5 mg/kg twice a day for four consecutive days (B), and or six to seven years after the same exposure (C).

It seems that MDMA causes non-repairable damage, especially to serotonergic neurons, leading to degeneration of axons and loss of connections between cells.[9] These neurotoxic effects suggest that this drug is anything but innocuous. Though we're not exactly sure how regular or semi-regular recreational use affects the human brain, because these studies would require autopsies (and control groups!), in my view it doesn't look good.

For instance, the extent of MDMA use in humans is positively correlated with the decrease in serotonergic function.

A study published by Lynn Taurah and her colleagues in 2014 should be read by everyone thinking of using this drug.[10] The aim of their study was to see whether MDMA produces lasting effects on humans, as it does in other animals. Loss of serotonin and norepinephrine function would be especially predicted to produce depression, impulsivity, and cognitive impairment because serotonin transmission is so critically involved in mood, behavioral regulation, and thinking. Their study included almost a thousand subjects, about 20 percent drug naive and the remainder about equally divided among five separate groups of recreational drug users. One group used only alcohol and/or nicotine, another used cannabis, perhaps with alcohol and/or nicotine, a third had never used MDMA but had used amphetamine, cocaine, heroin, and/or ketamine. The last two groups used MDMA; the first had used the drug at some point during the previous six months, but not for at least three weeks, and the final group were former ecstasy users, who'd been abstinent for *at least four years*. The researchers assessed a variety of measures including several associated with mood and cognition. There were two major findings. First, former and current ecstasy users were virtually identical, and, second, these groups showed significantly more clinically relevant levels of depression, impulsiveness, poor sleep, and memory impairment. Again, these were recreational users, many had not taken the drug for years, and still deficits were strikingly evident.

Anecdotally, my interactions with users of MDMA match the findings of Taurah and her colleagues. The first user I knew well was a former undergraduate student named Doug. Incredibly bright and outgoing, he was eager to get research experience and worked in my laboratory one summer. Although he became less reliable as the weeks wore on, he made up for his spurious presence by offering clever and insightful ideas about experimental design and interpretation, and when he was on, he was really very good. I eventually learned that the reason for his spotty contributions was that he was working as a DJ at raves in a nearby town. This was probably in the late 1990s and a fairly new thing at the time. He was a good mixer and shared that MDMA helped him stay in the groove for the many hours of partying. After that summer, Doug's grades slipped a bit, but I didn't have much interaction with him until he asked to do research with me again the following summer. I wasn't thrilled, but because conducting research as an undergraduate was pivotal in my trajectory, I tend to do what I can to provide opportunities and gave him a spot. It didn't go well. He was all over the place with his ideas, made as many mistakes the first week as most newbies make in a semester, and couldn't remember what we'd discussed from hour to hour, let alone day to day. He apologized profusely and often, but I simply couldn't let him stay in the lab because we were working with live animals (mice) and their well-being is of both scientific and moral concern. By this time, we both recognized his dramatic slip, and even talked about the probable cause, because he offered that he might have done "too much molly." I bumped into him a few years later while I was attending a scientific meeting in the same town in which he worked as a bartender. More recently, I learned that a persistent state of chronic despair drove him to suicide.

Many researchers are ringing bells of alarm, predicting an increase in ecstasy-related psychopathology over the next decades. However, others are advocating for clinical testing of MDMA for treatment of psychological disorders, especially trauma-related disorders. The private organization called MAPS (Multidisciplinary Association for Psychedelic Studies) recently received FDA approval to study MDMA as an adjunct to therapy for PTSD. It posits that MDMA's ability to increase feelings of trust and compassion toward others will prove useful and that pure MDMA taken a limited number of times in moderate doses will be safe. It's spending about $25 million aiming to have an approved prescription medicine by 2021, noting that for-profit pharmaceutical companies are not interested in developing MDMA into a medicine, perhaps because its patent has expired, or perhaps to avoid future liability.

I feel as if this book were full of doom and gloom, but in a way this may be the most depressing chapter (no pun intended). Every drug that acts on the central nervous system to change the way we feel will cause an opponent process. For most drugs discussed in this book, it's likely that with abstinence the *b process* will dissipate and the brain return somewhere near its nascent state. Unfortunately, it doesn't look as if this is going to be the case with stimulants, and particularly for those abusing amphetamines or ecstasy. As discussed, coke, meth, and E interact not with receptors but with transporters, but that in itself is not what makes them dangerous. Indeed, selective serotonin reuptake inhibitors as well as older tricyclic antidepressants are some of the most well-known transporter-blocking drugs, and neither shows evidence of permanent brain damage. Even cocaine doesn't appear to cause the same sort of long-term damage that amphetamines and ecstasy do, perhaps because it—like the antidepressants—stays in the synaptic gap rather than being transported into cells like its more toxic cousins. It seems likely that the presence of these drugs inside the nerve terminals somehow accounts for their toxic effects.

Ecstasy is the epitome of the irony inherent in the opponent process. While rolling, users experience a sense of deep okayness, seeing the best in themselves and those around them. As a result of this positive bias, they are accepting of things and people, including themselves, just as they are in all their stunning beauty. But the ensuing damage ensures the opposite experience: a sense of alienation and despair. It seems no coincidence that the popularity of this drug rose with more fragmentation and disconnection in present-day society. We hardly know our neighbors and, at least in the United States, spend much of our day isolated from our communities, including the natural world, as we drive around in metal boxes and spend our days and nights interacting with machines. This is painful and unnatural, but is the antidote a drug that temporarily lifts the veil to show us ourselves in each other, and then strengthens the walls between?

+ + +

8

Seeing Clearly Now: Psychedelics

Purple haze all in my brain,
Lately things don't seem the same

—Jimi Hendrix, "Purple Haze" (1967)

Good Science

There are countless substances that alter perception, some more potently than others. Because of this similarity in effect, some experts include substances like MDMA, ketamine, belladonna, and salvinorin A in a catchall category with drugs like LSD, psilocybin, mescaline, and DMT. However, the mechanisms by which these drugs affect the brain, their specific effects, and their behavioral consequences including addictive liability differ so widely that it seems appropriate to parse more finely. Though some researchers would disagree with my classification, this chapter is devoted exclusively to a narrow group of mind-opening drugs that all act in the same way, by activating a particular type of serotonin receptor, to modify experience. I'll call these psychedelics. I'll use the term "hallucinogen" for compounds that induce hallucinations but are not primarily serotonin 2A receptor agonists and cover those later.

A singular fact about psychedelics is that the majority of scientists who study abused substances don't think these are addictive. Though highly regulated across the globe, the compounds LSD, mescaline, DMT, and psilocybin are certainly much less harmful than many other substances and may even confer benefit. Despite political and social opposition and a dearth of research (due to regulatory constraints), the scientific community remains curious about the effects of these compounds and open-minded concerning the potential therapeutic benefit they may afford.

The recent history of these drugs began with the isolation of mescaline in 1898 by the German chemist Arthur Heffter, who obtained peyote from a colleague in the United States. About a decade earlier, Parke, Davis & Co. in Detroit had received caps or "buttons" from peyote cacti from an unknown source in Texas who was apparently curious about what the chemists could discover. The company sent some of these to Germany, to Louis Lewin, considered a founder in the field of psychopharmacology. Professor Lewin was taken enough by peyote's psychochemistry to travel to the American Southwest the following year and start his own collection, surely no trivial matter at the time, and became Heffter's source. Heffter was eventually able to isolate and characterize several pure alkaloids from the plant and, using both animal experiments and "self-experiments" and testing them one at a time, showed that mescaline was the chemical responsible for peyote's profound psychoactive properties. Although ingesting the topic of your research is frowned on as a strategy in labora-

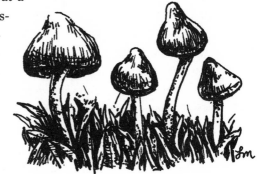

tories today, Heffter recognized early that aside from studies of toxicology, animal models aren't especially useful in characterizing pharmacological effects of psychedelic drugs. As a result of Heffter's experiments, mescaline was eventually synthesized by Ernst Späth in 1919, paving the way for studies of its clinical effects in the early part of that century.

Psilocybin, mescaline, and DMT are natural compounds that have been used for millennia by indigenous people in sacred rituals; LSD is a synthetic compound, created by Albert Hofmann, a Swiss chemist, in 1938. He inadvertently ingested a small amount five years later, in 1943, to make a life-changing discovery that he famously described, in part, as an "uninterrupted stream of fantastic pictures, extraordinary shapes with intense kaleidoscopic play of colors." He tried it again three days later, and many times thereafter, continuing to take small doses throughout much of his life and promoting what he saw as its "sacred" value as an aid to the "mystical experience of a deeper, comprehensive reality." He simplified this description later, calling it "medicine for the soul."[1]

In an interview with Stanislav Grof, he defended this view in the face of LSD's reputation as a dangerous party drug:

GROF: Usually, when you read the psychedelic literature there is a distinction being made between the so-called natural psychedelics, such as psilocybin, psilocin, mescaline, harmaline, or ibogaine [sic], which are produced by various plants (and this applies even more to psychedelic plants themselves) and synthetic psychedelics that are artificially produced in the laboratory. And LSD, which is semi-synthetic and thus a substance that was produced in the laboratory, is usually included among the latter. I understand that you have a very different feeling about it.

HOFMANN: Yes. When I discovered lysergic acid amides in ololiuqui [the seeds of a flowering vine], I realized that LSD is really just a small chemical modification of a very old sacred drug of Mexico. LSD belongs, therefore, by its chemical structure and by its activity, in the group of the magic plants of Mesoamerica. It does not occur in nature as such, but it represents just a small chemical variation of natural material. Therefore, it belongs to this group as a chemical and also, of course, because of its effect and its spiritual potential. The use of LSD in the drug scene can thus be seen as a profanation of a sacred substance. And this profanation is the reason that LSD has not had beneficial effects in the drug scene. In many instances, it actually produced terrifying and deleterious effects instead of beneficial effects, because of misuse, because it was a profanation. It should have been subjected to the same taboos and the same reverence the Indians had toward these substances. If that approach had been transferred to LSD, LSD would never have had such a bad reputation.[2]

Hofmann makes several critical points. First, that LSD belongs in a class with other so-called sacred drugs used by indigenous people. Use of these substances, like virtually all psychoactive drugs, began in community groups employing them for social, spiritual, and medicinal purposes. Indigenous people all over the world took advantage of their local pharmacopoeia to explore the meaning of their own existence; they did this in ritualistic settings, with shamans or teachers as guides. It's hard to know exactly how and when these "trips" began, but they were certainly well before people began recording history. However, there are some very ancient artistic depictions. Stone paintings in the North African Sahara suggest that aboriginal tribes were eating psychedelic mushrooms as early as 7000 B.C. Paintings in Spain date a bit later. Mescaline has been used for at least fifty-seven hundred years in the region of Mexico and western South America, obtained from several species of cacti including peyote, San Pedro, and Peruvian torch. Ayahuasca, which contains DMT, has long been used in Peru and other parts of South America.

Hofmann next complains about the drug culture's irresponsible use of LSD (of which I admit I'm an example). He's not the only one to make this point. Theodore Roszak, who coined the word "counterculture" and chronicled the hippie movement, noted in 1969,

> Perhaps the drug experience bears significant fruit when rooted in the soil of a mature and cultivated mind. But the experience has, all of a sudden, been laid hold of by a generation of youngsters who are pathetically a-cultural and who often bring nothing to the experience but a vacuous yearning. They have, in adolescent rebellion, thrown off the corrupted culture of their elders and, along with that soiled bath water, the very body of the Western heritage at best, in favor of exotic traditions they only marginally understand; at worst, in favor of an introspective chaos in which the seventeen or eighteen years of their unformed lives float like atoms in a void.

Harsh, but probably true. Like other good things, the drug might have been "wasted on the young." However the most fundamental point Hofmann is making is that psychedelic use may benefit humanity. He said this many times and many ways throughout the course of his illustrious career as a scientist and author, including at a speech at his centenarian celebration, where he said, "It gave me an inner joy, an open mindedness, a gratefulness, open eyes and an internal sensitivity for the miracles of creation. . . . I think that in human evolution it has never been as necessary to have this substance LSD. It is just a tool to turn us into what we are supposed to be."[3]

As we'll see, I tend to agree.

Distinctions

Lysergic acid diethylamide, or LSD, compared with its natural analogs, psilocybin, N,N-dimethyltryptamine (DMT), and mescaline, differs most in its potency. LSD is one of the most potent psychoactive compounds we know and is effective at about two hundred times lower concentrations than the next strongest, which isn't much different from the rest. Only 50 to 100 micrograms (0.00005 grams = 50 micrograms) of LSD, usually delivered through a paper tab that has been dosed with a small amount of liquid, will induce a trip that lasts for six to twelve hours. Mescaline is similarly long acting, while psilocybin's duration is about half as long. All of these are typically taken orally and induce rapid and profound tolerance. In fact, besides the fact that they don't cause dopamine release in the nucleus accumbens, this tolerance is so quick that regular use is pointless.

DMT has a much shorter duration of action and when smoked, as is typical for recreational users, a very rapid onset. This has led to its reputation as a "businessman's trip" because it lasts only about the length of a short office break—about five to fifteen minutes. However, DMT effects can last a few hours when the drug is ingested along with another compound that blocks the enzyme monoamine oxidase (MAO), which is necessary to prevent the natural breakdown of DMT in the digestive system. One source of such an MAO inhibitor is the ayahuasca vine, *Banisteriopsis caapi*. A sacramental drink brewed from this vine and the leaves of a DMT-containing plant (typically *Psychotria viridis,* but there are at least fifty other species of plants, as well as three sources from mammals and one from a particular species of sea fan) has been used historically in religious and healing rituals and, increasingly, by tourists. There is a booming "ayahuasca" industry in South America as thousands of people a year tramp to the Amazonian rain forest for insight. DMT is reported to produce vivid mystical experiences, euphoria, and hallucinations especially of geometric forms, higher intelligences, extraterrestrials, elves, and God. It's illegal in most countries and has several structural analogs including 5-MeO-DMT, which is slightly more potent. DMT is Schedule I in the United States, although some religious groups have permission to use the drug for ceremonial purposes.

I have no experience with DMT, which is also available in synthetic form, but have tried the others (LSD, psilocybin, mescaline). I don't recall seeing any elves, but if I did, I'm sure they were friendly. The first time I tripped, and every time after, was like opening a door into a much more vast and mysterious existence than the one I usually inhabited. Twenty or thirty minutes after I put a tab under my tongue, chewed a peyote button, or ate magic mushrooms, a delicious feeling of invitation, crumbling boundaries, and mind-bending joy would begin to bubble up from deep inside me. Though I never had a bad trip, I did have some that were very intense and not entirely pleasant, but the ride was always so interesting to my scientific mind that wherever it took me seemed well worthwhile. My good fortune was probably partly due to my optimistic constitution and the somewhat idiotic naïveté that characterized the 1980s.

Taking these drugs is like taking a trip to an unknown place, by a vehicle that is not in your control, to have encounters, also beyond your control, that are significantly outside anything you know. Though I suppose it's not comfortable for anyone to feel a loss of control, I'm probably more inclined than the average person to relish the sense of being swept away from solid ground, both because I tend to seek novelty and thrills and perhaps because of a deep-seated urge to touch the ineffable. In retrospect, I see my experience with psychedelics as the antithesis of my use of stimulants, where I knew exactly where I was going and how to get there, without distraction.

Acid trips helped me realize at a critical time in my psychosocial development that I was not the center of anything. What a relief! Also, and perhaps because I was temporarily freed from my egocentric delusion, I became more aware of an ever-present, infinite, and wonder-full energy in, and around, and through, every speck of creation. Though I can't summon it as intensely as when I was tripping, that feeling has stayed with me. Because of their lasting halo, I tend to agree with Hofmann and others that psychedelics are a tool for the path but not themselves a path. To think otherwise is like mistaking the finger pointing at the moon for the moon itself.

My experiences were typical, in that psychedelic "trips" are characterized by intense emotions and mystical realizations, along with (mostly visual) hallucinations. In addition to a tendency to perceive everything as infused with a vital energy, one sees, for example, solid surfaces that seem to reveal their vibrational atomic nature, or trees that bend and ripple as if they were made of fluid; there is often a sense of oceanic oneness and increased connectedness with others and the rest of the world. However, there are also "bad trips," which are equally profound but sometimes psychologically and spiritually challenging, which is why the drugs have a reputation of being very unpredictable. These vary tremendously, as do the positive experiences. Like dreams, they reflect relatively unconstrained and unfiltered activity in the cerebral cortex. One friend I was tripping with at the beach became convinced that the ocean was boiling (it *was* a hot day) and saw his legs melting into the sand as he concluded we were all doomed; another saw lizards being birthed from a pizza and then the walls of her dorm room. Letting go of the illusion of control and even embracing the experience (what *would* it be like to melt?) are the strategies that worked best for me. On the other hand, even bad trips are often perceived positively in retrospect, as a way for the user to face challenging concepts, such as the eventuality of his own mortality, or to make other difficult existential realizations. This contrasts sharply with the sorts of adverse experiences caused by other classes of drugs. A drunken stupor combined with physical retching, for instance, is never seen as a good thing, nor is the disconnection from perceptions while under the influence of dissociative anesthetics, a subject of the next chapter.

All of these higher-order effects, along with the fact that non-human animals generally don't choose to self-administer these drugs, have made it difficult to characterize the pharmacodynamics of psychedelics. The discoverers, you may remember, learned about the structural-functional relationship by using themselves as test subjects. As a side note, I was struck while reading the early literature that the single exception to humans being the sole species to show any interest in volunteering to test psychedelics were nonhuman primates who—only when deprived of normal external stimulation, including social interactions—would sometimes prefer to sit alone in their cages and self-administer psychedelics, lost in what, I can only imagine.

Experienced

The despair of beginning to realize that my neural wiring somehow precluded regular social use of drugs was bad enough, but the thought of never doing *any* drugs was too much to bear. Some I could take or leave. Like oxygen, I took alcohol for granted, benefiting from its properties but not caring all that deeply. My emotional tie to most other substances was similarly agnostic, though by the time I did my last shitty line of coke, I wished never to see the stuff again. On the other hand, my relationship with weed and psychedelics was full of deep feeling. My grief at having to quit smoking pot took many years to get over, but honestly, I couldn't imagine staying off the acid bus. Though instructed in the "day at a time" philosophy and able to apply it to most substances—even marijuana, because deep down I knew my smoking was mostly to quell the panic and boredom of not smoking—I found staying away from psychedelics forever an especially crushing blow. In fact, deep in my heart I've held on to the notion that I might be able to drop acid for special occasions, fully realizing that the LSD itself would make any occasion special.

I've often been caught in this logical koan: I can do any drug I want, as long as I don't really want to do it. The converse, which seems equally tragic, is that those who can afford to use are the least deserving candidates. My husband is one of these; when he has a rough day, I'll suggest he have a drink, and he just looks at me blankly. He often leaves beers unfinished or turns them down at a concert because he's too far from the aisle to make regular bathroom visits. I can't begin to comprehend the sort of reasoning that he practices, because I'd readily risk not being able to get out of the parking lot.

But I've held out hope for psychedelics. A few years ago, clean and sober for dozens of years, I floated my fantasy with a close group of friends. Because they are mostly neuroscience naive, I launched into an elaborate justification of why this class of drugs was unlike the others and in fact should not be classified as addictive. These drugs don't lead to the release of dopamine in the nucleus accumbens (need I say more?), so nonhuman animals won't self-administer them. They can't be taken compulsively, because tolerance is so fast and profound that it precludes regular use; there's not a whit of evidence for dependence and no compelling evidence for harm in most people. Finally, I topped all this off with the seemingly solid argument that a brief dip into the stream might be just the thing to propel me out of my several-year psychic jam. (Middle age can be described as the "mean time" between the glorious power and innocence of youth and the wisdom and freedom of the more seasoned, and I was eager to move it along.) My friends just laughed, and I could tell by my childish frustration at their inability to appreciate my rationale that my plans—at least for the time being—were sunk.

The light at the end of the midlife tunnel seems visible to me now, and I'm in a better place than I was when I made the appeal to my friends. For now, adopting the same strategy I take with most drugs, I haven't picked up since 1986, though neither have I closed the door. This is partly because I'm inclined to do exactly what anyone—even I—tells me I can't, so making rules about behavior doesn't work very well in my case. And it is partly because I acknowledge that I benefited from psychedelics, but also that the returns on repeated doses were diminishing. My takeaway from psychedelics is the light they shone on what is always available but somehow usually obscured. Having understood a bit about my place in the cosmos—Infinitesimal! Glorious!—and about the cosmos itself—Replete! Glorious!—I feel it would be immature to continue returning to the teat. This in itself should speak to the nonaddictive nature of these drugs, because having had the full benefit of experience never stopped me before.

Medicine

It's a shame Albert Hofmann didn't live just a few more years because it now seems quite probable that his hopes for psychedelic drugs—as aids to living better—may be realized soon.

Over the past several years, small clinical trials have suggested benefits of psychedelics for depression, alcohol and nicotine addiction, and end-of-life anxiety.[4] The studies have taken place at reputable medical schools such as Johns Hopkins, New York University, and the Imperial College in London and are very carefully conducted and monitored. Most of the research so far has used psilocybin, partly because the shorter, three-hour or so, trips are more amenable to laboratory visits, but one employed LSD, and the U.S. Food and Drug Administration recently approved a protocol for the first trial of ayahuasca as a treatment for depression. The necessary plants are being grown in Hawaii to be ready for the start of the study about the time this book is published.

Some of the most provocative studies have been those treating patients diagnosed with terminal illnesses.[5] These typically involve dose-controlled ingestion of a psychedelic compound in an enhanced clinical setting, often looking like a nice hotel room supplied with a good sound system through which facilitative music is played. (If this sounds like the "acid tests" of Haight-Ashbury in the 1960s, I can understand

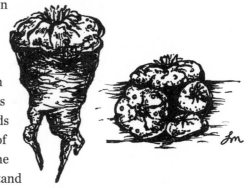

why, but the major difference is tight control over the dosing and the presence of trained clinical personnel.) Participants usually have two several-hour sessions of guided tripping, separated by a few weeks to a month. The clinical guides help patients process the experience safely during the several hours of deep introspection. When they emerge, these patients often report newfound insights. The guides also encourage patients to continue to explore significant insights after the visits are over. Terminal patients undergoing psilocybin-assisted therapy report greater acceptance and decreased depression and anxiety about dying.

These studies are preliminary, but it's important to keep in mind that we have no better alternatives to offer people suffering with the thought of imminent death. Anxiety, depression, and addiction are rampant in part because the existing treatments aren't sufficient, and of course we are all going to die. So far there have been no adverse side effects in this second generation of studies (there are equivocal reports of a few negative experiences in studies that occurred in the first wave), and many participants seem truly moved by the experience.

Correlational studies are also intriguing. Though correlational studies can't assess cause-and-effect relationships, they help us understand whether variables are related to each other. One recent report assessed the potential benefits of the insight enabled by these drugs for pro-social behavior.[6] Researchers led by Professor Peter Hendricks at the University of Alabama found about a 25 percent decreased likelihood of theft or other property crime, and an 18 percent decreased likelihood for violent crime, in those who used psychedelics among almost half a million U.S. adults who participated in the National Survey on Drug Use and Health between 2002 and 2014. Interestingly, use of other drugs including cocaine, heroin, marijuana, and MDMA were all associated with *increased* risk for committing these crimes, suggesting that the benefit is specific to psychedelic substances. Along similar lines, another group used an experimental design to study the influence of psilocybin on a wide range of psychological measures associated with pro-social behaviors. Participants were assigned to a control group that received placebo or one of two experimental groups that both got psilocybin but varied in the amount of instructional guidance they received about daily spiritual practices such as meditation in order to see whether this helped augment any drug effect. There were twenty-five participants in each group, and subjects came for the same procedure twice about a month apart. In addition to showing that the treatment was safe and enjoyable, follow-up interviews six months later showed lasting benefits of the drug on several measures including altruistic behavior, increased spirituality, and an improved sense of well-being/life satisfaction.[7] These findings replicate and extend previous research, reviewed in depth by David E. Nichols. For example, José Carlos Bouso and colleagues compared more than a hundred regular ayahuasca users with actively religious matched controls on a number of psychological variables including well-being, cognition, and several indices of psychopathology.[8] Ayahuasca users were lower on all psychopathology scales, including tendencies toward OCD, anxiety, hostility, paranoia, and depression. They demonstrated no difference in cognitive measures but scored higher on measures of psychosocial well-being than a control group of religious subjects who did not use psychedelics.

So how might these drugs be working to help alleviate persistent depression, reduce addictions, enable people to face their own deaths with aplomb, and enhance pro-social behaviors? That question is still being answered, but a recent review suggests that it is via their specific interactions with one of the serotonin receptors (the serotonin 2A).[9] The drugs induce activity in genes that are associated with neuroplasticity and disrupt established/default connections between groups of neurons, which "may allow the brain to re-enter a state of widespread global plasticity, whereby the maladaptive patterns responsible for the manifestation of psychiatric illness can be reset."[10]

It is still too early to know definitively exactly how the drugs interact in the brain to produce their effects, or tell whether benefits will be substantial and lasting, but the future for researchers studying these substances looks brighter than it has in decades. A millennia-long history of medicinal use in humans, coupled with anecdotes of life-changing experiences, and now these encouraging preliminary empirical findings suggest that we may be on the cusp of a more humane way to treat psychopathology. Who wouldn't be open to the possibility of effective treatment for the epidemics of depression, anxiety, or antisocial personality disorder, especially one that costs less and seems to have fewer side effects than existing pharmacotherapies?

9

A Will and a Way: Other Abused Drugs

> I mean, that's at least in part why I
> ingested chemical waste—it was a kind
> of desire to abbreviate myself. . . . I
> wanted to be less, so I took more—
> simple as that.
>
> —Carrie Fisher, *Wishful Drinking* (2008)

Won't Stop Us Now

When I was just starting to experiment with drugs, there was an urban myth that smoking banana peels would get you high. I tried it, along with hyperventilating, and taking aspirin and cola, in my first clumsy attempts to mess with my mind. I don't know if these specific superstitions endure, but I am sure I'm not the only one to attempt such pointless exercises.

The drive to alter experience is universal. We have been intentionally administering substances in order to alter psychological functioning as far back as we have written records (and likely before). For every advance in our understanding of how the brain works, we discover that there exists a natural product to exploit it. Plants make morphine, cocaine, nicotine, caffeine, marijuana, and a plethora of hallucinogenic compounds naturally, and these substances have been used since at least the beginning of the archaeological record. Alcohol was first brewed about ten thousand years ago in the form of mead from fermented honey and has been popular ever since. The recreational and/or ritualistic use of chemicals has occurred in every human population with the capacity to avail itself of drugs.

Nor is drug taking a solely human activity. Countless other species, from other primates to insects, appear to appreciate chemical-induced changes in experience. Most of us have seen cats enjoying the effects of catnip, but many animals eat opiates, and alcohol from fermented fruit is popular among mammals, birds, and insects. One of my favorite examples from the animal kingdom comes from a particular species of ants (*Lasius flavus*) that fosters beetles (*Lomechusa*) in an apparently symbiotic relationship where the ants feed adult beetles and nurture their larvae (at the expense of their own colony) in order to regularly partake of a goo exuded from beetle glands that seemingly serves no purpose other than to make the ants *really* calm. The universality of drug taking across the animal kingdom has suggested to some that such activity may reflect a biological drive, like that for food or sex.

This chapter will cover a wide range of drugs from different classes, including some naturally derived from plants or animals, as well as a large and growing collection of synthetic compounds. Some of these substances are very harmful, and others less so, but for any drug administered regularly, we've seen by now, there is compensatory adaptation on the part of the brain, and therefore the risk of addiction.

And Still More Stimulants

We've already spoken about the most well-known stimulants including nicotine, cocaine, methamphetamine, and ecstasy,

despite evidence of a high incidence of dangerous reactions in users. Eventually, science prevailed and ephedra-containing dietary supplements were made illegal in the United States. (Sales of products containing ephedra extract but not containing ephedrine, the active ingredient, remain legal.) Ephedrine is also regulated because it can be used to synthesize methamphetamine. A related popular over-the-counter medication with similar side effects is pseudoephedrine. Pseudoephedrine is the active ingredient in nasal decongestants, such as Sudafed. It is no longer freely available on the shelves of U.S. pharmacies, because it too can be used to make methamphetamine.

All of these drugs act in a similar way by blocking reuptake of catecholamines (a subset of monoamines that are distinguished by having a chemical structure that includes a catechol ring) including dopamine, norepinephrine, and epinephrine. Excess dopamine is thought to underlie the euphoric effects, while flooding synapses with norepinephrine makes a person more alert, and the rise in epinephrine contributes to peripheral effects like stimulating heart rate and blood pressure. The compound fenethylline (also spelled "phenethylline" and "fenetylline"), and "marketed" under the trade name Captagon, has a slightly different pharmacological profile. The drug was synthesized in Germany in the 1960s and is a combination of our old friend amphetamine and theophylline, the natural stimulant found in tea. Until recently, it wasn't clear what accounted for the action of Captagon, but researchers have now determined that the drug's pharmacological and behavioral profile is the result of a functional synergy between theophylline and amphetamine.[1] The addition of theophylline enhances amphetamine's effects. The researchers used a novel and clever method to prove this by employing antibodies against different aspects of the original chemical as well as its breakdown products, and one of the side benefits of this research might be a vaccine against the drug. Because antibodies are so specific, such a formulation would make Captagon moot but likely precipitate more clandestine drug development because it wouldn't do anything to diminish the demand for uppers in general.

However, a vaccine could be useful because there is a huge black market for Captagon. The drug is heavily abused, especially (for now) throughout the Middle East, where it is popular with college students, and about 40 percent of users become addicted. Syria is a major producer of the drug, which has two main purposes in the country. First, it gives militants physical energy, alert nervous systems, and perhaps an inflated sense of confidence, which are all useful effects for waging war. Soldiers interviewed in a BBC Arabic documentary said, "I felt like I own the world" and "There was no fear anymore after I took Captagon." The other benefit is that sales help fund such warfare.

Take Me Away

Phencyclidine and ketamine are two examples of the class of drugs known as dissociative anesthetics. Phencyclidine may be more familiar as PCP or angel dust, and ketamine has been "marketed" as Special K, Kit Kat, or cat Valium. PCP was first developed as an anesthetic agent with less risk of overdose than the barbiturates. It did seem relatively safe at first, but it soon became obvious that the drug wasn't producing the deep state of relaxed unconsciousness resulting from typical (barbiturate) anesthesia. Though subjects weren't responsive and seemed to be breathing okay, they were also in an odd, trancelike, or catatonic state. Moreover, their muscles weren't flaccid as they would be when knocked out by a sedative-hypnotic, but seemed toned as if they were awake, though their eyes were open but vacant. The drug was used clinically for a few years, and though it did have a much higher therapeutic index than classic anesthetics, reflecting a very low risk of overdose, reports of problems began to develop. Some patients became agitated on the table; others were quiet but woke with postoperative reactions like blurred vision, hallucinations, dizziness, or aggressive behavior. It was abandoned for clinical use in 1965 but found its way to the streets in just a couple of years. In the meantime, Parke, Davis chemists made many analogs in the hope of finding something with shorter duration and less potential for delirium. One of these safer alternatives was ketamine. Ketamine became a successful anesthetic and is still often used in humans, especially during pediatric and geriatric surgery, where the risk of overdose from barbiturates is higher, or when there isn't time for delivering and monitoring barbiturates, such as on a battlefield. Ketamine is also widely used in veterinary clinics and marketed as Ketaset, Ketalar, and Vetalar.

One of the ways to assess anesthesia, or unconsciousness, is by looking at neural activity using an electroencephalogram, or EEG. High-frequency waves, like very choppy water, indicate arousal, but as we go into a state of relaxation, and then deeper and deeper stages of sleep, the EEG shows slower and slower waveforms—like the big sweeping West Coast swells attractive to surfers. This happens as the neurons' activity becomes more and more synchronous, driven no longer by what's happening in our environments but instead by deep subcortical structures applying their own rhythm. The peculiar EEG pattern generated under these drugs looks like a mix of complex waveforms, suggesting to researchers a dissociation of sensory and limbic systems, or sensing and feeling. In fact, the EEG tracings mirror the class's name—dissociative anesthetics. These work by producing a state of separation between sensation and "self." In addition to this sense of detachment, sometimes accompanied by a feeling of leaving one's body, the drugs produce amnesia, so whatever happens under their influence is lost to conscious memory.

After it was dropped from the clinic, PCP was readopted, surprisingly, by countercultural, antiwar types and dubbed Peace Pill. That reputation didn't last long, though, and in a few years the drug spread across the country, mostly known as angel dust. By 1965, illicit use had reached epidemic proportions, such that in some cities, including Washington, D.C., there were more psychiatric admissions due to toxic reactions to PCP than for alcohol abuse and schizophrenia combined. Schizophrenia is not a totally unfounded comparison, because to hospital workers the effects of too much "dust" looked similar to some symptoms of this disorder: hallucinations, distorted perceptions of body shape, size, or material (for example, feeling as if one were made of rubber or plastic), and losing track of time. In addition, at least some of PCP's effects are due to increased levels of the neurotransmitter glutamate, and excess glutamate has also been implicated in schizophrenia. The effects just described don't sound especially pleasurable, but there are other cognitive changes that users seem to enjoy more, including having meaningful insights or visions of supernatural beings, though afterward these experiences are fuzzy to say the least.

These drugs block the flow of ions through one of the glutamate receptors, known as the NMDA receptor. NMDA receptors are widely distributed throughout the brain and play a critical role in many functions including cognition and memory formation. Glutamate signaling also influences many other transmitter systems, so again, as in most cases, connecting the psychological effects with the neural actions isn't entirely straightforward. While some pleasurable sensations may arise via direct actions on glutamate signaling, there is ample evidence that the drug also potently stimulates mesolimbic dopamine neurons: dopamine levels rise in the nucleus accumbens following systemic administration, drug-naive volunteers roundly seem to like the drug and desire more, and given the opportunity, experimental animals will readily self-administer these drugs. These experiments present an odd picture, as you can imagine, because subjects lose the ability to control their body position. Nonetheless, most manage to prop themselves up and somehow activate the lever that will deliver the drug.

Though neither of these drugs is especially popular, ketamine has a committed following by a subset of recreational users. Unfortunately for them, chronic use is bad for the brain. Reflecting the ubiquitous role of glutamate signaling, a variety of negative effects are evident in regular users, supported by parallel research in other animals, including problems with incontinence, cognitive deficits, gross abnormalities in brain structure, deficits in dopamine signaling, and a loss of both dopamine and glutamate synapses. Because these drugs are still used in the clinic, there is some concern, especially regarding pediatric anesthesia, that they may be altering brain structure and function, although studies in humans are so far inconclusive.[2]

Unwittingly, many people probably have a similar drug in their medicine cabinets. Dextromethorphan is a cough suppressant found in many "DM" formulations. These have been on the market for many years, at first in pill form, but because that was too easy to abuse, the drug companies decided to put DM in syrup, thinking that having to choke down the contents of whole bottles at one time would dissuade abuse. Users need about twenty times the normal dosage to achieve the desired effects of impaired balance, euphoria, and visual hallucinations.

Not surprisingly, swallowing down the sweet, sticky fluid is a small price to pay for some especially motivated adolescents. However, cough syrup contains more than the drug of choice, and users may also be consuming huge doses of expectorants or antihistamines, both of which produce unwanted side effects. To counteract this, enterprising entrepreneurs came up with a way to extract the substance from cough syrup and offer it for resale, often on the internet. Between 2000 and 2010, DM abuse more than doubled, and though it is not currently scheduled, the DEA has listed it as a drug of concern.

One Good Bush

About nine hundred species of mint-like shrubs make up the very large genus *Salvia*. The name *Salvia* comes from a Latin word meaning "to heal." There are three main branches of *Salvia:* the largest is found in Central and South America, with approximately five hundred species; another in central Asia and the Mediterranean has about half that number; and one in eastern Asia has around a hundred species. Given this incredible diversity, it's perhaps not surprising that at least one species turns out to have psychoactive properties.

Salvia divinorum is a small perennial shrub, native to the southern Mexican state of Oaxaca. Indigenous use involved either mixing juices extracted from the leaves, crushing them with water to make a tea, or chewing and swallowing a large number of fresh leaves. Any of these methods make the effects come on more slowly than smoking, generally over a period of ten to twenty minutes, but the experience also lasts longer, from about thirty minutes up to one and a half hours. Smoking is the preferred method for most recreational users, because it provides a much faster, more intense (but briefer) high, usually beginning within a minute and peaking in five to ten minutes before gradually diminishing. The hallucinogenic effects include uncontrollable laughter, vivid, rapidly changing visions including abstract moving forms, "out of body" experiences, synesthesia, a mixing of senses, and a shifting sense of "self."

Though the effects sound somewhat similar to classic psychedelics, a survey of people in a position to compare the two classes of drugs found that less than 18 percent described the effects as similar.[3] The main active ingredient in the salvia plant is salvinorin A, and this compound has a unique pharmacological profile that still has scientists puzzling. As it turns out, salvinorin A is the most potent natural hallucinogen so far discovered (LSD surpasses it, but this, of course, is synthetic).

Salvia has been used for a long time in religious rituals by the Mazatec people. It seems an incredible coincidence that this plant grew in the same area as and was used by the same community that practiced spiritual medicine with psilocybin-containing mushrooms. Salvia was also used by the Mazatec people for various medicinal purposes such as treating diarrhea, headaches, and rheumatism.

Though it is a potent hallucinogen, the active ingredient of *Salvia divinorum*, salvinorin A, is not grouped with the other psychedelics in my taxonomy because the drug's mechanism of action is totally different. Pharmacologists are at least as excited about the compound salvinorin A as are recreational users. Until its characterization, no other molecule with a similar structural-functional profile was known, so it has opened up a new avenue of research. Salvinorin A is a naturally occurring, potent, and selective kappa opioid agonist. Kappa receptors are one of the canonical opioid receptors, often appreciated best for anti-opioid effects. Kappa receptors don't interact well with morphine or other narcotics, and we'd thought that activation of kappa receptors produces a dysphoric state. For instance, kappa activation has been implicated in the miserable feelings associated with alcohol withdrawal.[4] Salvinorin A has no other known activity across fifty other receptors, transporters, and ion channels, including the serotonin 2A receptor—the principal site of activity of classic psychedelics such as LSD and psilocybin.[5] So far, so mysterious.

Another way salvinorin A differs from psychedelics is that it appears to have abuse liability. Though initial reports suggested that the drug decreased dopamine levels in the accumbens and produced an aversive state, those turned out to be evident at much higher doses than recreational users seek and obtain.[6] A more recent comprehensive assessment of the drug's reinforcing effects in rats, using doses analogous to those of human users (for example, 0.1–10 micrograms per kilogram of body weight), found just the opposite: animals will work to obtain the drug, they form positive associations with contexts in which the drug is delivered, and most convincingly, salvinorin A increases dopamine levels in the nucleus accumbens.[7]

This unique pharmacology—that is, activating kappa opioid receptors and increasing mesolimbic dopamine—is not well understood. Therefore, though we don't yet have information on the effects of repeated use, and in particular what adaptation might occur at kappa opioid receptors or other compensatory sites, salvinorin A appears to be a drug that would lead to addiction. At present, salvia is not illegal in the United States, according to federal law, but the DEA lists it as a drug of concern, and about half the states, as well as many countries, have enacted legislation prohibiting its sale and use.

Cooking

I once had a friend, Laurie, who'd been clean a couple of years when she called to report that she'd found a great new product called Spice. She excitedly reported it was natural. (Why do some people think this means safe? Anthrax, mercury, radon, and about a zillion other toxic compounds are natural!) But according to everything she could learn on the product's packaging and a quick internet search, Spice was also harmless. Laurie was especially confident about its safety because it could be purchased so easily—at most gas stations. Eventually, she ended up at the hospital incoherent and with slurred speech and, after she came to, acknowledged the stuff was probably not a "free lunch."

Spice is shredded plant material combined with synthetic cannabinoids that work by mimicking THC. These concoctions first appeared in the early twenty-first century as a "legal" form of marijuana, sold under the name K2 and/or Spice. Like bath salts, Spice is often labeled "Not for Human Consumption" and disguised as incense. Therefore, it was not until late 2008 that Spice products were investigated for their psychoactive properties by the European Monitoring Centre for Drugs and Drug Addiction and a couple of years later came to the attention of the DEA following a tremendous spike in usage and toxicity reports. Because the chemicals used in Spice have a high potential for abuse and no medical benefit, the DEA has since made many of the active chemicals illegal.

However, the development of new synthetic cannabinoids has remained ahead of the legislative scheduling process and continues to diversify more quickly than laws can be passed and forensics can detect. Multiple structural classes of synthetic cannabinoids have been developed, including at least 150 unique compounds. In addition to evading regulatory laws, individual users appreciate these compounds because they are usually able to avoid detection in standardized drug testing—a particular benefit for military personnel or people subject to urinalysis by the legal system or employers. Like marijuana, the effects are variable: some users report anxiety, others relaxation, some have hallucinations or paranoia, others not. In general, though, the high is more intense than that associated with marijuana, because the synthetic versions of THC are usually much more potent agonists at the CB_1 receptor.

The risks also seem greater. A number of clinical case studies have documented markedly greater toxicity following an acute use of Spice than marijuana, across a broad range of physiology including gastrointestinal, neurological, cardiovascular, and renal systems. These effects have recently been reviewed by Paul Prather and colleagues.[8] Most alarming are reports that acute toxicity from Spice can result in death, likely due to its strong pro-convulsant effects.

Another major area of concern has to do with the association between cannabinoids and psychosis. There is a well-established positive correlation between exposure to weed or other natural cannabinoids and a diagnosis of schizophrenia. The general consensus has been that cannabinoids don't cause the disorder but can unmask a latent vulnerability, bringing schizophrenic symptoms to the surface that might otherwise have remained below the threshold for detection. In contrast to earlier models of the disease, researchers now see it as an expression of a number of interactive and complex factors, much like the way we view addictions. In this view, all sorts of things can influence risk including a biological predisposition but also living under stressful conditions and, apparently, excessive activation of CB_1 signaling. Rapidly accumulating reports of acute and lasting psychosis elicited by use of synthetic cannabinoids are raising alarms. Acute use of Spice can bring about psychosis-like symptoms of paranoia, disorganized behavior, violent behavior, visual and auditory hallucinations, and suicidal thoughts, which seem to persist much longer than more typical cannabinoid effects. Interestingly, many of these effects are seen in users with no other evident risks for psychosis and schizophrenia. The drugs are so new, that evidence for a causal relationship between Spice use and psychosis is hampered by the fact that the literature consists entirely of case reports. Almost all synthetic cannabinoids studied to date bind more tightly to CB_1 receptors than THC does. This increased potency is naturally associated with more robust tolerance, dependence, and withdrawal, caused by a dramatic drop in the number of functional CB_1 receptors. In such cases, users can expect profound cross-tolerance so that smoking weed would actually be about as effective as smoking the grass in your backyard. It may be the case that users are getting this message, or that they've had adverse effects themselves, because rates of use of Spice seem to have peaked. According to the National Institute on Drug Abuse, reported use among twelfth graders dropped from 11.4 percent in 2011 to 3.5 percent in 2016.

Making It Simpler

GHB (gamma hydroxybutyrate; marketed as Xyrem) is a central nervous system depressant and also a metabolite of the inhibitory neurotransmitter GABA. Therefore, it is naturally produced in the brain, though in small amounts, much lower than those used and abused recreationally. When GHB was first developed in the laboratory in 1964, it was intended for anesthetic purposes, and also tested as a pain reliever, but not pursued by drug companies at that time due to high incidence of seizures and vomiting. The drug more or less disappeared until the 1980s, when it was marketed and sold as a supplement to promote muscle growth for athletes and bodybuilders. However, by

1990 there were so many reports of GHB-related toxicity that the FDA declared the drug unsafe and banned over-the-counter sales. It was listed as Schedule I in 2000 and classified as a Class C drug under the Misuse of Drugs Act (1971) in the U.K. in 2003; it is now controlled across all EU member states. However, GHB use continued to grow, especially as a "club drug," along with ketamine and Rohypnol (flunitrazepam; a benzodiazepine that also produces profound amnesic effects). These drugs are popular at dance parties because their effects are similar to those produced by alcohol, but without the hangover. Surveys carried out in the U.K. of a self-selected group of 3,873 clubbers suggested rates as high as 15–20 percent, but general use is much lower. In a European School Survey conducted in twenty-five European countries in 2003, only 0.5–1.4 percent of fifteen- to sixteen-year-olds reported that they had ever used GHB.

About twenty minutes following administration, which is usually oral, the GHB user experiences varying effects that depend on the dosage, mood, and particular circumstances. On the upside, users commonly experience an increase in energy, stamina, and sensuality. They feel euphoric, happy, relaxed, and sexually enhanced. On the downside, GHB users also typically experience loss of muscle coordination, headaches, nausea, drowsiness, difficulty concentrating, amnesia, dizziness, difficulty breathing, and vomiting. At high doses, GHB use may result in sedation, decreased heart rate, loss of self-control, slurred speech, seizures, inability to move, coma, and even death. The GHB high often lasts up to four hours but may be extended when used with other, similar drugs.

GHB appears to produce much of its behavioral effect via its action at $GABA_B$ receptors. Structurally these receptors are very different from $GABA_A$ receptors, and we are still not certain how GHB's interactions with the receptor lead to behavioral effects.

The drug also has effects on dopamine signaling as well as other neurotransmitters, including serotonin and norepinephrine. Using it over a long period leads to the development of tolerance and dependence. This dependence can be so profound that some users consume the drug every couple of hours around the clock to avoid withdrawal symptoms.[9] The clinical features of GHB withdrawal are similar to those seen with ethanol and/or benzodiazepine withdrawal except that they begin earlier, typically within a few hours of the last dose and are very severe at the twenty-four-hour mark, a reflection of the fact that the drug is metabolized quickly. The most commonly seen features of withdrawal include tremor, irregular heartbeat, anxiety and agitation, hallucinations, delirium, sweating, hypertension, and confusion. Although seizures appear to be less common than with ethanol withdrawal, delirium, agitation, and other neuropsychiatric signs appear to be more common and more marked in patients withdrawing from GHB. GHB dependence is best treated with high-dose benzodiazepines, or barbiturates in those who are tolerant to benzodiazepines.

There did ultimately turn out to be a medical use for the drug, and getting approval was quite controversial because it was already classified Schedule I and still is. Nonetheless, the drug *was* approved by the Food and Drug Administration in 2002 for use in the treatment of narcolepsy (a sleep disorder). GHB is a successful treatment for these patients who have disrupted nighttime sleep, excessive daytime sleepiness, and cataplexy—sudden loss of muscle control that is usually triggered by a strong emotion such as anger or frustration. All three of these symptoms are significantly reduced by GHB. To get approval, the company had to agree to a unique risk management program called the Xyrem Success Program, designed to be sure the drug was only used by narcoleptic patients and not diverted to other people. There is a patient registry monitored by the FDA, and only for these people the DEA considers the prescription version a Schedule III drug, meaning it can be prescribed with refills as long as a DEA number is listed on the prescription. To prevent misuse, a central pharmacy dispenses the drug and mandates use of a specific prescription form to verify the physician's familiarity with the medication.

Really Desperate

Inhalant abuse remains the least studied form of substance abuse and refers to the intentional inhalation of vapors from commercial products or specific chemical agents to achieve intoxication. Inhalants are a diverse class of substances, usually easily found in our everyday environments, and most commonly used by people who are unable to secure either more expensive or less readily available sources of a "high." There are literally hundreds of commercially available products, containing single substances or mixtures, that can produce intoxication if inhaled.[10]

Solvents like nail polish remover, glue, ink in pens and markers, gasoline, shoe polish, and paint thinners are easy to obtain and inexpensive. Aerosols from spray cans are another source, like those used to hold vegetable oils for cooking, deodorants, and spray paints. Gases, including propane, butane lighters, and the ever-popular nitrous oxide, provide yet more opportunities for sniffing. All these drugs produce euphoric effects. Nitrites like amyl nitrite (poppers) and butyl nitrite are also inhaled but primarily used to heighten sexual arousal—almost like a really transient Viagra—by relaxing muscles and dilating blood vessels.

Effects occur rapidly and are short-lived, although some abusers repeatedly or continuously self-administer inhalants to maintain a preferred level of intoxication.[11] Experimenting with these drugs is very popular; most inhalant users begin as children and discontinue use quickly, so these are the only substances used by young people where use peaks in preadolescence and tends to drop off through the teen years. While this isn't the case for everyone, and continued inhalant abuse is a serious concern, the biggest danger is that users are at increased risk for getting involved in other harmful substance use.[12]

Although inhalant abuse exists worldwide, it's especially common among the poor and the homeless, including especially children who work or live on the street. Because these chemicals are so prevalent and often free, they have wide appeal for people who feel powerless and are seeking a way to escape a harsh reality. In some poorer communities and among Native American people, use can be much higher. For example, in São Paulo, Brazil, nearly 24 percent of nine- to eighteen-year-olds living in poverty had tried inhalants, and over 60 percent of youth were found to use inhalants in several Native communities in the United States and Canada.

In addition to their easy access, these drugs are appealing because the high happens very quickly. Inhalants are rapidly absorbed from the lungs into the bloodstream and quickly enter the brain, where they depress CNS function—sometimes by enhancing inhibitory activity at $GABA_A$ receptors, and sometimes by inhibiting excitatory activity in glutamate or acetylcholine pathways. There are also general effects on electrical currents by poorly understood direct actions on ion channels. The effects of inhalants are similar to getting drunk, but some people report experiencing something like hallucinations. A sudden sniffing death syndrome may occur, but more commonly these compounds tend to damage the liver, kidneys, lungs, and bone in addition to the brain. Repeated use has been linked to cognitive impairment, likely due to degeneration of neural pathways as the axons that conduct information throughout the brain lose function, and perhaps to lead poisoning from huffing gasoline. There is also evidence of cerebellar dysfunction and damage to peripheral nerves, effects that may impair movement. Death can also occur from heart attack, choking on vomit after falling unconscious, or other injuries, such as suffocating on plastic bags. Like alcohol, inhalants can have profound effects on the developing fetus, including severe and permanent cognitive deficits.

Summing It Up

Many of the synthetic drugs got their feet off the ground by slipping past regulatory commissions, often as close analogs of other controlled or illegal substances. In 1986, the same year I got clean, the Federal Analogue Act was passed to help deal with the flood of synthetic drugs coming from backyard chemists or overseas suppliers hoping to exploit and share the benefits of known compounds by making small modifications and remarketing the substances as something new. Before 1986, it was the case that each new compound had to have its structure fully characterized before it could be made illegal, so producers would race to develop variants of illegal compounds that retained (or improved upon) psychoactive properties before federal commissions could outlaw them. By the late 1980s, though, the writing was fully on the wall, and compounds with structures "substantially similar" to other Schedule I or II substances were made illegal by analogy. The need for this law was so compellingly obvious, even to Congress, that it was introduced, passed by both houses, and signed by the president of the United States (Reagan) in less than two months. However, like virtually all legal attempts to control the drive to use drugs, it hasn't made a dent.

+ + +

10

Why Me?

Every time I draw a clean breath,
I'm like a fish out of water.

—Narcotics Anonymous

Four or Five Reasons

As I first began to consider the starkest of choices (*never* again?),
the question rose as inescapably as GI activity anticipating a shot
of cocaine: "Why me?" There seemed plenty of reasons that I
shouldn't be one of those people who couldn't control their use.
I thought I was smarter . . . or more resolute . . . or more deserving. Besides, I was just getting started and way too young to have
a habit. My desperate evasions were just like those of millions
of other people determined that they'd never be like a drunkard
parent or a panhandling nomad; not one of us sees it coming.

Questionnaires available to help with self-diagnosis ask, "Do
you drink more than you intend to?" "Do you frequently have
more than 4–5 drinks a day?" (to this I have known many people
to say no, only to eventually admit that they mixed their drinks
in tumblers), and "Has alcohol caused you problems at home
or work?" The imprecision and subjectivity of questions such
as these are not lost on most addicts, especially because one of
the classic symptoms is denial. Almost by definition, we're more

inclined to think of our use as the solution to our troubles than the cause. Sure, I met some of the criteria some of the time, but my ability to fool teachers, clinicians, and law enforcement stemmed from an ability to fool myself.

It's not unusual to rail against fate, especially when faced with a fatal diagnosis, but the thoughts and feelings that I experienced had the particular flavor of someone who'd co-authored her dilemma; cognitive dissonance is a big part of the denial engine. What this means is that when behavior and cognition don't jibe, the expeditious solution is to change our mind: Why would I hurt myself? (Because that makes no sense) I must not be hurting myself.

But eventually, when there was finally nothing left but to face the truth, I felt fury, shame, and betrayal. It seemed supremely unfair that I, who loved mind-altering substances more than anything or anyone, should have this problem! Moreover, why have to face such a brutal ultimatum when I was young, rather than in my forties? At least at that ripe old age, my reasoning went, sobering up might not be such a terrible drag. But as I gradually came to terms with the fact that I didn't use drugs as much as they used me, my thoughts turned to figuring out why on the way to fixing it.

It wasn't as if my behavior was so outside the norm. Practically everyone I knew used chemicals. Why didn't substances get the best of them? The girl I was thrown out of ninth grade with, for example, was well on her way to a successful career and a happy home life when I landed in the treatment center. We seemed to start off on the same road, so it didn't seem right that I was the one to veer into a ditch, while she coasted down what looked to be easy street. In fact, the world seemed full of people who were having their cake and eating it too. My family, friends, and co-workers all drank, and many used other drugs, but somehow they didn't end up trading themselves for one last bump, hocking the family jewels, or wrapping vehicles around poles. Streets and clubs worldwide are filled with users enjoying themselves—happy and just a little blitzed. How to explain the fact that only a subset of us pursue this path all the way to an early grave?

My desire to understand why reflected a need to explain what otherwise seemed an inexplicable failure of my deepest self. I was hardly unique in this. Millions of people on the planet want to understand the mess they or their loved ones are in. Hundreds of scientists working today have spent their entire careers studying addiction; therapists and teachers of other kinds strive to treat the illness. The scope of suffering is so broad and so deep that the possibility of effective treatment, let alone a cure, is a holy grail for much of humanity. The quest is now at a polar opposite of the moral perspective that characterized understanding a century ago. At that time, convention held that addiction resulted from a weak character. When people asked why those like me didn't simply show some discipline or moderation by adopting more rational choices, it seemed reasonable to conclude that they must simply be morally weak. Predictably, in the age of the brain, the pendulum has swung far to the opposite pole: morality, character, and personal responsibility are moot; addicts are victims of an abnormal biology, and "choice" may itself be an illusion. The good news, we are told, is that medicine will soon find a cure.

So, in the end, why me? After about thirty years of highly motivated focus on the research, I'd say there are four primary reasons people like me develop addictions. Well, actually five, but I'm saving the gloomy news for last. The four are these: an inherited biological disposition, copious drug exposure, particularly during adolescence, and a catalyzing environment.

It's not necessary to have all four, but once some threshold is reached, it's like breaching a dam—virtually impossible to rebuild. So, with enough exposure to any addictive drug, any one of us will develop the hallmarks of addiction: tolerance, dependence, and craving. But if the biological predisposition is very high, or use starts during adolescence, or certain risk factors are present, less exposure will do the trick.

Genetics

An inherited risk for addiction was demonstrated as early as the mid-twentieth century, though of course people recognized much earlier that addiction tends to run in families. But speaking Slovenian also runs in families, and that isn't inherited, so how do we know there is a biological predisposition? There are two main sources of evidence. The first is that the more DNA one shares with an addict, the higher one's risk. Typical siblings share 50 percent of their DNA, but identical twins share virtually all of it, and they are about twice as likely to have similar addiction histories. Second, if the biological child of an addicted individual is adopted immediately after birth by a family with no history of addiction, he or she retains an elevated risk, as of course do unadopted children of addicts or alcoholics, though obviously they are also subject to more risky environments in addition to the biological risk.

Let's say what you inherit is like a deck of cards: red cards make it more likely to develop a problem, and black cards are protective; high numbers and face cards have a larger influence than do small numbers. Everyone gets dealt a hand, and the genetic risk is reflected by the balance of red and black and the value of these cards. This may seem straightforward, but I've left out an important caveat: your "hand" comprises thousands of cards, and many of these are barely consequential or entirely inconsequential. Moreover, the mix of risky and protective genes combines with each other and aspects of family history and the current environment to confer liability. The problem has been likened to finding particular straws of hay in an entire field. Or like locating a nameless building in an unknown city, but you're not sure which country it might be in.

A common strategy is to start with what we know about how drugs interact with the brain and work backward. This "candidate gene" approach has suggested that genes that code for processes associated with neurotransmission by dopamine, acetylcholine, endorphin, GABA, and serotonin may be associated with disordered drug use, but the catch is that even when an association has been proven, it fails to explain very much of the inherited risk; typical genetic findings account for a minute fraction of the differential risk among individuals. So, for instance, some people might have a tendency toward anxiety or be naturally endorphin deficient, and both of these states can be remedied by drinking. Those with a proclivity toward stimulant use may be partly so because they are unconsciously self-medicating an undiagnosed or subclinical deficit in the capacity to maintain focus and attention, due to alterations in dopamine transmission. Though these hypotheses seem plausible, and have some evidence to support them, such explanations neither account for the majority of substance use disorders nor can predict any individual's disease state. They may be part of the explanation but are nowhere near all of it.

Inherited information like this is largely conveyed by our genes, which are specific sequences of nucleotides (*a*denine, *t*hymine, *g*uanine, and *c*ytosine) made of deoxyribonucleic acids, better known as DNA. The DNA code is used to direct the synthesis of proteins, of which we are made, so a particular strand of DNA might instruct the cell to form muscle, hair, or the enzyme that synthesizes dopamine. Most of our DNA is identical to that of all other humans—we all make dopamine in the same way, by specific enzymes transforming the amino acid tyrosine—but a subset of our genes are polymorphic, which means they exist in more than one form. Many of these polymorphisms are substitutions in a single nucleotide, akin to replacing a letter in this chapter. Though such a small alteration doesn't seem as if it could have a measurable effect, even a single nucleotide change in a gene may result in a small structural modification in the product, thereby altering its function. Other polymorphisms are more substantial, such as insertions or deletions of whole chunks of DNA, but evolution caps the amount of difference, because too much change is usually lethal to an embryo. Over the past decades, thousands of research hours have been spent trying to find the minute modifications that predict susceptibility to disordered drug use.

This hasn't gone as well as we'd hoped, and we still don't know what accounts for the vast majority of innate risk. Scant few genes have been reliably associated with addiction liability, in part because, other than a polymorphism in a gene that codes for liver enzymes that help to metabolize alcohol, we have found no snippets of DNA that have a major impact on addiction. Instead of "genes for addiction," we have discovered dozens of locations on the genome where polymorphisms combine and interact to influence risk, and each variation in sequence may explain only a very small fraction (typically less than 1 percent) of the carrier's inherited liability. And there is no smoking gun, no sequence variation present in all addicts but not in social users. In other words, if you took a thousand hardened addicts and a thousand "normies" and compared their DNA—and this has been done repeatedly, believe me—there are no deterministic differences: most of the DNA is identical, and even when we get lucky and find that a particular sequence is more common in one group than other, there are plenty in the other group with the sequence too. In such a case, the variation is simply present at a higher frequency in addicts or "normals," and obviously such a pattern doesn't enable us to predict an individual's outcome. Moreover, a particular strand of DNA may be present in only a subset of those possessing what appears to be the same disorder—for instance, a stimulant addiction. These realities make it very difficult to locate influential genes.

Nonetheless, sometimes the less focused studies comparing genomes of addicts with those who don't struggle yield "hits" that lead to novel hypotheses. This is cool because such findings help us better understand how the brain works, but not terrific in that they tend to generate more questions than they answer. Such sequences—often far from the genes that seem related to core addiction processes—may make us more or less likely to respond to our environment in particular ways, and this adds another layer of complexity, as if the site of culprit "houses" we are hoping to locate depends on conditions, like the weather or time of day. All genetic influence, we've learned, is context dependent and incredibly complex.

Epigenetics

Open-mindedness and humility are necessary attributes of any good scientist, and as Carl Sagan noted, "in science it often happens that scientists say, 'my position is mistaken,' and then they . . . actually change their minds."[1] It took cloning our genome, yet still mostly failing to link genes to addictive behavior, for us to appreciate how overly simplistic our view of the hereditary units had been. We assumed that breaking the genetic code would result in a fairly straightforward path to prevention and treatment, but in fact very little has been explained, let alone cured. Part of this may be due to the fact that we inherit more than a sequence of DNA from our ancestors: the double helix of spiraling nucleotides carries another set of instructions that are also passed down. This code consists of epigenetic—literally, on top of DNA—modifications that regulate the activity of the DNA and constitute a cellular memory of our ancestors' experiences. We now realize that epigenetic modifications overlaying the sequence of nucleotides, along with other indications of experience in the form of things like micro RNAs (which block RNA, the messenger that carries instructions from DNA), can have a big influence on which genes are translated into proteins, and when. Some addiction researchers think that these transgenerational modifications may account for the "missing inheritance"—that is, the genetic signature underlying the known heritability of addictive diseases.

The relatively new field of epigenetics is just getting under way, but it is thought that some of our parents' and grandparents' experiences are imprinted in our cells this way in order to adapt us for similar conditions. This is a good idea from a biological perspective, because the best index of the future is usually the past, and adapting well to our conditions is a primary example of biological fitness. For example, Rachel Yehuda and her colleagues have data suggesting that children of Holocaust survivors might carry epigenetic modifications from their parents that make them primed for stress.[2] Others have demonstrated that progeny from families enduring famine inherit a tendency toward metabolic thriftiness that predisposes them toward obesity.[3] As if, to err on the safe side, our DNA were prepared to help some of us carry a little extra cushion.

We're beginning to scratch the surface on how inherited

modifications to the DNA double helix contribute to complex traits like addiction, and data are accumulating to suggest that risk factors may be passed along epigenetically. When potential parents smoke marijuana, for instance, epigenetic changes could be priming subsequent generations for addiction. Conducting longitudinal studies in humans to identify such transgenerational impacts presents challenges, obviously. One of the biggest is that we can't randomly assign people to smoking and nonsmoking groups, so we can't rule out that those prone to smoking may possess tendencies to abuse other drugs as well. (This, again, was the main argument proffered by tobacco companies for decades: they argued that it was impossible to say that smoking *caused* cancer and suggested with surprisingly straight faces that those who smoked also coincidentally happened to be prone to metastases.)

In one experiment using nonhuman animals in order to assess for cause and effect, rats received eight exposures to a moderate dose of THC every third day across a twenty-one-day period during their adolescence, while a control group got the same regimen of placebo injections. The rats then grew up drug-free and reproduced—former partiers with former partiers, and abstainers with abstainers. When these rats' offspring grew up, those whose parents had THC as "teenagers" showed increased self-administration of opiates as well as behaviors associated with depression and anxiety.[4] In other words, the experiment suggested that if your parent used THC before you were conceived, you may be at increased risk for developing a mood disorder or an addiction. These studies are really just getting off the ground, but the robustness of the data is surprising even the scientists. And for a change, the blame isn't just focused on the mothers. Epigenetic marks through the paternal line are at least as profound, thought to be caused by small bits of RNA that accumulate in the epididymis, which is more or less the male version of the fallopian tube, and affect sperm on their way to the prize. Rapidly accumulating evidence along these lines has many scientists thinking that as a culture we are involved in a giant experiment. It's increasingly looking as if exposure to drugs of abuse in our parents and grandparents predisposes us to take drugs ourselves—effectively a *b process* across generations.

It's not impossible but seems improbable given what I know of my heritage that my addiction resulted from a parent's or a grandparent's experimentation with weed. But it's entirely plausible that other stressors played a part. Perhaps it was the stress that my grandmother experienced as she left home, barely an adult, to arrive by boat on Ellis Island, a relatively unempowered immigrant who worked as a maid before settling into an unhappy marriage and raising children with little support. Or perhaps it was a grandfather's heavy drinking, or the sadness my mother experienced in her own lonely marriage, or the relentless criticism my father endured and then handed down. Any or all of these might have biased me toward loneliness or alienation and predisposed me to find a way to escape.

This is the deeper story of inheritance. The sequence of nucleotides in each of our cells reflects our long human evolution as well as the particular history of our families, including both marriages and mutations, while the epigenome hovering above it "remembers" the experiences of our ancestors the way ruts in the road indicate where wheels have passed.

Early Exposure

Setting aside epigenetics for the moment, there is a large body of solid evidence that early exposure to marijuana causes changes in brain structure to embryos, children, and adolescents and that these structural changes can produce cognitive and behavioral deficits. There is also good evidence that exposure during development makes someone, among other things, permanently less sensitive to rewards, so that later, when given the ability to self-administer drugs of abuse, they take more.[5] Individuals exposed before they are conscious or making their own choices are set up for an addictive scenario.

For embryos or children exposed to drugs indirectly (through the placenta or secondhand smoke, for example), the effects are somewhat easier to parse, but for experimenting adolescents there is an additional layer of complexity: Is it the case that early use predisposes subsequent problems or that those who (perhaps for genetic reasons) are more likely to experiment as youth are also likely to become adults who use? In other words, is the early exposure causal or correlational? Maddeningly, the answer is yes: both are true. A predisposition to seek novel experiences, take risks, or escape pain, for example, may influence behavior across a lifetime, but we now also know that starting early, before the brain is mature, causes neural changes that foster problem use in adulthood. We call this the "gateway effect," and a growing body of research documents enhanced drug-taking and drug-seeking behavior in humans and animals following adolescent exposure to substances including cannabis.[6] These modifications are akin to those induced by prenatal exposure and occur basically for the same reason.

Developing brains are—by definition—primed to change. Everybody knows that kids learn more easily than adults, whose behavioral rigidity is explained by a relative reduction in neural plasticity. Compared with adults, kids are behaviorally more flexible, and their brains are much more malleable. The decade or so between puberty and brain maturation is a critical period of enhanced sensitivity to both internal and external stimuli. Notice how integrated the brain is with social development: by appreciating new ideas and experiences, teens develop a sense of personal identity from which important life choices follow. An explosion in neural rewiring underlies developmental milestones like affirming likes and dislikes, discovering and nurturing talents, and becoming a sentient individual separate from one's parents. In this way, experiences in adolescence are concretized by lasting patterns in the brain and behavior. The downside of this is that any neurobiological consequences of drug use are much more profound and longer lasting when exposure occurs during adolescence than when it occurs after about age twenty-five—the neural definition of adulthood.

The upshot is that starting so young had an exaggerated impact on my developmental path. It's likely that by pounding so hard on vulnerable neural circuits such as the mesolimbic pathway, I developed an insensitivity—the way listening to music that is too loud can make you hard of hearing. It's not that I can't feel pleasure; it just takes more volume to make an impression. This might help explain why such a significant portion of my income goes to airline tickets; traveling is one way I stimulate dopamine when daily life fails to do it. The flip side of this, also supported by strong evidence, is that the older one is when one begins getting high—on anything from alcohol to amphetamine—the less likely one's use is to become addictive.[7] It's likely that if I'd begun a little later, my trajectory wouldn't have been so precipitous. In fact, research indicates that most people with a substance use disorder started using during adolescence and met the criteria before age twenty-five.[8]

Unfortunately, this information is unlikely to prove a deterrent to young people. That is because adolescents' general tendency to explore and experiment (or more colloquially, "engage in reckless behavior") is partially due to underdevelopment of the prefrontal cortex. This region, right above the eyeballs, is most responsible for "adult" abilities, such as delay of reward, abstract reasoning (including statements like "*if* I spend the rent money on a zone bag, *then* . . ."), and impulse control. By some ill-timed developmental plan, the prefrontal cortex is the last brain region to reach its mature state. What's more, this area of the brain is one of the regions most affected by a substance use disorder. What a pickle!

Though it feels a bit like shouting into the wind, I've nonetheless implored my own children as well as my many students to carefully consider the evidence. Popular opinion, wishful thinking, or even favorable legislative policies are no substitute for data. The world's best science now indicates that the long-term consequences of adolescent drug use, acting upon a very plastic brain that is highly tuned to news and pleasure while at the same time a bit retarded in terms of self-control, may be grim. And not to put it all on the kids, adults also need to consider what influence *our* behavior could have on baby brains before we adopt drug policies and practices that subject future generations to the consequences.

Beyond the gateway effect, we know that chronic THC users have an increased tendency to feel blue, show more difficulty with complex reasoning, and suffer from things like anxiety, depression, and social problems. Scientists know that the relationship is at least partly causal: regular marijuana use leads to these pathologies.[9] For adults, the neural changes caused by marijuana may partially derail a successful and otherwise fulfilling life or hamper its development, but the good news is that such capacities would likely recover with abstinence. However, consequences are more likely to be permanent when exposure occurs during adolescence. In addition to dampening reward sensitivity, THC acts in pathways that ascribe value or import to our experiences, and if these are muted, especially for a lifetime, the impacts are likely to be broad and deep. The heart of the matter is that the brain adapts to any drug that alters its activity and it appears to do this permanently when exposure occurs during development. The more exposure to the substance we have, and the earlier we have it, the more strongly the brain adjusts.

An Addictive Personality

Taking a more "macro" view, one commonly hears someone described as having an addictive personality (personality tends to reflect inborn and persistent tendencies), and indeed there may be aspects of personality that incline a person to use, but as usual the relationship is not simple. For example, the gene encoding the serotonin reuptake transporter (the same one affected by MDMA and SSRI antidepressants) can be inherited in multiple versions. These versions differ in how quickly the transmitter is recycled, and this small kinetic alteration has been associated with differences in the tendency to act impulsively, engage in pro-social behavior, and respond to stress. However, this influence is largely contingent on the amount of early childhood nurturing or maltreatment. Serotonin activity also contributes to how anxious an individual tends to be, and anxiety is also shaped by relationships with our primary caregivers, for better or worse. Those with high anxiety—whether they got there from inherited liabilities or stressful experiences, or both—are obviously more likely to enjoy the benefits of sedatives like alcohol and benzodiazepines.

A similar profile exists for dopamine and an inclination toward risky behavior. Some of us naturally have more—or less—sensitivity in this system so that the ability of abused substances to stimulate dopamine pathways makes drugs more salient for some of us than for others. Before they even begin using, addicts are thought to have altered activity in their meso-limbic dopamine system, making it hypersensitive to possibility. One study found that risk taking was higher in eleven- to thirteen-year-olds with exaggerated sensitivity to reward and that this predisposition made it much more likely that they would be diagnosed with a substance use disorder four years later.[10] Dopamine sensitivity, like serotonin recycling speed, isn't an either-or trait, like blood type, but instead is normally distributed in the population. That makes it harder to investigate, and normally distributed tendencies are typically the product of multiple influences.

An appetite for risk is not just about drugs, either. Several groups of researchers have studied the relationship between mesolimbic dopamine and the financial risk assumed by traders. They find that those with more dopamine take higher risks, supporting the hypothesis that one's subjective impression of the potential value of an investment is greater with more dopamine. Moreover, impulsive and high-risk choices are more likely in other animals with higher mesolimbic dopamine including dogs, monkeys, and rodents. But "risk" doesn't fully capture the nuanced ways that dopamine neurotransmission contributes to behavior. In another study, subjects were given information about two possible travel destinations in two separate experimental sessions.[11] During one session they received a placebo, and during the other they received a drug that enhanced dopamine activity. Self-described expectations of a pleasurable vacation were higher for whichever destination was promoted while dopamine levels were enhanced, and subjects were more likely to choose this option because presumably it seemed more promising.

These findings suggest that natural variation in dopamine signaling contributes to differences in the way people respond to things they encounter in their environment, and in particular whether we feel tempted or tepid when exposed to the possibility of reward. The old view that equated dopamine with a feeling of pleasure is too simplistic. Rather, high dopamine tone correlates with enhanced sensitivity to potentially rewarding experiences, as if the message concerning something of potential value were being delivered at a higher volume and essentially drowning out drawbacks, as we might see in any person developing addiction including to drugs, but also when they are gambling or scheduling a vacation to a new spot.

The major point is that individual differences in our neurobiology make moderation more or less likely. The neurobiological playing field is not even. Natural differences in serotonin activity and mesolimbic dopamine, as well as other influential factors, have important implications. For some people, through birth, experience, or a combination of both, the appeal of drugs is greater than for others. I remember being awoken one morning by a friend from school who wanted to go windsurfing. As I got ready, I pulled a bottle of vodka out of the freezer and offered her a drink. She responded, "But it's 11:00 a.m.! You just woke up!" As far as I was concerned, she might as well have been discussing the price of papayas in Caracas. Another time, sober for several years, I was leaving a party along with a colleague who had had only two beers. Her rationale included the time of night and having to work the next morning, along with a few other facts that also seemed entirely irrelevant. Even today, I'm confounded by people who can drink or use other drugs but don't. For me, and others like me, nothing short of impending doom (and often even that) would provide enough incentive to forgo pharmacological stimulation. People who stop after only one drink, mete out cocaine like a banker, or keep a bag of weed around for months are entirely foreign to my experience and beyond my capacity to comprehend.

On the other hand, I am able to relate to the depravity in this story from the Associated Press: "Man Accused of Trying to Swap Baby for Beer." Apparently, someone called the police after this man offered her a three-month-old baby in exchange for two forty-ounce beers. I'm sad to say that I really do understand the perversion of values that enables such an insane proposal, and while responsibility has to be attributed to the addict, it seems obvious that no person in what might be called a "right mind" would do such a thing.

The Lesson of Firewater

The business of DNA—making new structures—is a daily one. When we wake up, circadian genes stimulate arousal, activity, and hunger; a stressful encounter activates genes that direct the synthesis of hormones to help us meet challenges; and learning new things, perhaps like the material in this book, induces a proliferation of synapses that are the basis of long-term memories—even in adults, because we all retain some plasticity until the day we die. Some gene activation is purely transient, like that reflecting our daily rhythm, while other activation is long lasting, but the basic fact is that our DNA is exquisitely tuned to the environment. Vast swaths of nonprotein-coding DNA, making up about 98 percent of the genome, are sensitive to an unending stream of environmental input and translate these signals to affect gene transcription. That is, they use stimuli such as nurturing by a parent, the contents of our meals, a roller-coaster ride, or a difficult interaction with a boss to guide suppression or enhancement of protein synthesis, orchestrating a symphony of molecular changes that plays from a score of everything we experience—what's in the air, in the news, the background and foreground of our lives.

So, what type of environmental input paves the way for addiction? It is impossible to provide an exhaustive list because the universe of possible influences is virtually limitless. However, many of the known contributors are obvious ones, such as family stress, childhood abuse or neglect, environments with few positive role models, or a general lack of opportunity. These factors are not only vague but hard to quantify: What family doesn't experience stress? How much stress is too much? While we're at it, stress itself is so nebulous—something we all know but somehow can't quite define—making it hard to characterize its predisposing influence. These factors also tend to cluster: as might be expected, a stressful or unstable family environment increases the chance for addiction. Women, in particular, are likely to abuse substances in an attempt to self-medicate traumatic experiences such as sexual or physical abuse.[12] Economic status, family stability, religiosity, and education have also been identified as aspects of our environment that can contribute to, or protect from, a tendency toward disordered use.

Understanding environmental influences has been helped somewhat by twin and adoption studies. As mentioned earlier, even monozygotic clones (that is, identical twins) who share 100 percent of their DNA, not to mention many early experiences, have only about a 50 percent chance of having addiction in common, which is more than fraternal twins, but about half that needed to conclude that genes alone are responsible. Other than the obvious culprits like those listed above, thousands of studies suggest that random environmental influences—mostly too unpredictable and inscrutable to even be picked up by our experimental methods (for example, a particularly stressful day in middle school)—play an important role. Despite the potential for data overload, some researchers (with top-notch math skills, I might add) spend their careers trying to parse environmental influences that are even more dense than the information found inside our cells.

In graduate school, I had my perspective enlarged when I took a course on Native American history and culture and chose to write my final paper on the very high rates of alcoholism in this group. At the time, I shared the dominant view that Native Americans possessed a faulty gene or enzyme or some other aspect of brain circuitry that was responsible for decimating the indigenous population. I figured I'd spend some time in the library perusing the literature and summarize the causes for an easy A.

Native Americans happen to have the highest rate of alcohol use disorders of all ethnic groups in the United States, blighting entire communities in incalculable ways. For example, on some reservations close to half of children are born with fetal alcohol poisoning, and rates of addiction are similarly through the roof. Because all drugs of abuse use the placenta as a freeway, where they often have permanent effects on fetal brain development, high rates of alcohol use have devastating impacts that are perpetuated through generations. Alcohol is especially problematic because its effects are most potent early in development, often before someone even knows she is pregnant.

I launched into research databases and catalogs full of naive enthusiasm that soon turned to wonder and then to disbelief. Not only was I frustrated by a dearth of good review papers, but there was not much to review. This is not to say that there were no studies. In fact, there were loads of them: investigations of genes, neurochemicals and structures, brain wave patterns, liver enzymes . . . you name it. Tons of effort had been spent trying to identify the unfortunate constitutional factor that renders these people—already given a short stick, if one at all—so helpless under alcohol's influence. There wasn't one.

As I confronted my own assumptions, I realized how incredibly convenient a biological explanation for Native addiction rates would be for the rest of us. If we could attribute the epidemic of alcoholism and fetal alcohol effects on reservations to something about "them," we wouldn't have to ask about our complicity in the systematic denigration of their cultures, the theft of land and other resources, or realize that being exiled with little hope for personal growth or community prosperity might drive anyone to drink.

I should be careful to note that I am not saying there are no biological differences between Native Americans and other cultural groups. In fact, small differences in ancestry are maintained or magnified as people partner with others who share their background. However, no biological differences have been discovered that explain the higher rate of addiction in these people.

So, if not biology, what could be the source of all the car accidents, cirrhosis, damaged children and families in Native American communities? The plain answer is lots of drinking. Few of us spend much time on reservations. Only when I studied them did I realize that other than partaking in the endless font of cheap booze, there's not much else to do. Though specific sets of genes or epigenetic tags may someday be found to account for some of the blight, there are a lot of powerful and definitive contributors right under our noses, including high rates of poverty and unemployment and a scarcity of opportunities in general.

Though the conditions most of us live in aren't as dire, situational factors—often part of the fabric of our lives and therefore particularly easy to overlook—contribute to every person's choices. Who and what we encounter on a daily basis, including our relationships, workplaces, neighborhoods, media, and opportunities, all weigh in to influence who we are and what we become.

Faulty Reasoning

So for the last time, why me? The short answer, despite considerable time and effort, is I don't know. It's likely that my innate tendencies formed from dozens of risky nucleotide sequences and as many or more epigenetic marks worked with avid and early use and other environmental influences to load the dice in such a way that I am more likely than most to die from substance overuse. The important final factor is implied in that "worked with" because each of these influences has a direct effect on my outcome but also affects each other, forming a web of complex interactions. So, while I can elaborate on science's lack of a definitive explanation almost indefinitely, the bottom line is that there are likely as many pathways to becoming an addict as there are addicts.

Science is frustrating and rewarding for exactly the same reason. The more closely we examine any aspect of reality, the more we see how much there is to learn. Complexity, ambiguity, and contingencies are the rule in all of nature. One of my favorite aphorisms reframes the dilemma by suggesting that the aim of science is not to open a door to infinite wisdom but rather to set a limit on infinite ignorance. As a result of looking closely at any problem, we increasingly realize the flaws in our assumptions and ask better and better questions. So, I can say with absolute certainty that there's not "a gene" for addiction, nor is it caused by a "moral weakness"; it doesn't "skip a generation"; all people aren't equally vulnerable, nor is any one person equally at risk across the life span. In other words, we know a lot about the causes of addiction, and they are complicated.

Here is another disappointing fact related to the limits of science. Because final proof is so elusive, researchers work with probabilities. While families and clinicians want to explain the causes of a disorder within individuals—why is she this way?—science focuses on proclivities within the whole population. What this means is that despite all we know, we are unable to declare with certainty which individuals will or will not develop an addiction. Instead, research suggests that the likelihood is higher or lower in some groups than in others (that is, those with addiction, depression, or anxiety in their immediate family, those with little opportunity for self-improvement, and so on). In other words, not "will I" but "how much more likely am I" to become an alcoholic if my parent or grandparent lost control of his or her drinking than if no one in my immediate family had done so? The answer is about 40 and 20 percent, respectively, versus 5 percent. In other words, I can't precisely say why my use spiraled away from anything like an acceptable pattern, but I can point to factors that probably contributed.

Underlying all this uncertainty is the reality that we still have no objective measure to use for addiction. In fact, the National Institutes of Health can't even settle on a name for whatever it is people like me have. We've used "addict" or "alcoholic" and then "drug dependent"; now we talk about having a drug use disorder. Changing names or diagnostic criteria in the *Diagnostic and Statistical Manual of Mental Disorders* (also known as the *DSM,* currently in its fifth edition) might provide some with an illusion of progress, but I think it just makes it more clear how little we truly understand.

11

Solving Addiction

Do not weep; do not wax indignant.
Understand.

—Spinoza (1632–1677)

Just a Baby

The rise of neuroscience has been fueled by the promise of explaining the seemingly inexplicable complexities inherent in human behavior. At the start of the modern era, the neurophysiologist and philosopher Sir John Eccles made the case that "better understanding of the brain is certain to lead man to a richer comprehension both of himself, of his fellow man, and of society, and in fact of the whole world with its problems."[1] Sir John died in 1997, and I'm not sure how he would now reinterpret the optimistic projections he made at the peak of his career. On the one hand, we've had astounding leaps in brain science over the past fifty years. We've learned about how genes influence the structure and function of the brain; have developed an impressive array of snazzy techniques to visualize neural substrates, their connections, and their activity states—even in awake and autonomous subjects; and have a variety of ways to engineer genetic changes we want to achieve. The particular focus of Eccles's own studies, the synaptic gap between nerve cells, has offered up a font of revolutionary insights, and this knowledge has been a springboard for drug development. It's hard to appreciate just how far we've come until we realize that about the time he wrote that statement, brain scans were reserved only for extreme cases because they required injection of either air or opaque dye before taking a standard X-ray; MRI and CT scans were still more than a decade away.

On the other hand, while our tools have advanced, and our questions are becoming more and more sophisticated, it's still worth asking whether all the neurohype has paid off. Especially if you suffer from a behavioral malady, the answer is, unfortunately, no. The bitter fact is that almost without exception one's chance of cure from any chronic brain-related disorder is more or less the same as it has always been. Despite massive efforts, Alzheimer's disease, mono- or bipolar depression, schizophrenia, and addictions still lack a causal explanation, as well as any effective cure. This surprises many people, perhaps because we have a bias toward news of significant findings rather than a view of the broader landscape that is characterized mostly by 2 steps forward and 1.99 back. Bottom line: despite small advances in understanding addiction, rates of addictive disorders are increasing.

Still, it is important to remember that in comparison to astronomy or physics the field of neuroscience is a neonate. About a hundred years ago, the field of astrophysics knew much more than it does today. How can this be? At the time, scientists were quite certain they knew the size and structure of the universe. Of course, this was before they had the foggiest notion about quantum mechanics, string theory, dark matter, or other paradigm shifts stemming from empirical research. In fact, astrophysics today barely resembles the field as it was in the early twentieth century. Space physicists these days are much more aware of what they don't understand than they were then.

We could characterize the change as a reduction in certainty and a rise in humility. This was a very good thing for the field, not only because it more accurately reflects reality, but also because a stance of openness and questioning is a catalyst to more discovery. No one is going to learn what they don't want to know.

Enthusiasm and excitement around the new field of neuroscience have perhaps led us to overstate what we know at this juncture. Like the field in general, I was lacking humility about the incredible complexity of the nervous system when I embarked on my quest to cure the disease of addiction. When, either by some oversight of the admissions committee at the University of Colorado or by an outright miracle, I got to graduate school, right from the start things didn't go well. In fact, not a single experiment in my first year and a half panned out. Seven years later, it was finally dawning on me that I'd be lucky to explain even a facet of addiction. Yet when I left Boulder in the mid-1990s for a postdoctoral fellowship in Portland to work with experts in behavioral genetics, I somehow thought this area would be simpler. I planned to switch gears away from studying the role of stress and learning, in order to map the genes underlying addiction. It seemed a fortuitous time and place to be involved in such an endeavor, in part because of the broad commitment to gene mapping, including the Human Genome Project (HGP).

The aim of the HGP was to clone all human genes. In other words, as a result of this ambitious group project, everyone would have access to the nucleotide sequence of the genome. The medical promise appeared tremendous. In possession of the DNA code, many assumed that identifying causes and developing cures would be relatively trivial. Because we knew that disorders like bipolar, anxiety, and addiction run in families, it seemed straightforward to compare the genomes of affected individuals with those that were not and identify rotten pearls in the strand. Boy, were we ever mistaken!

Published in 2000, the human genome has been useful, but mostly not in the way we'd expected. Our first wake-up call was that the number of human genes turned out to be much, much lower than anyone anticipated. Because we assumed that human complexity was based in genetics, and because, though our evolutionary history is no richer than that of, for example, potatoes, our culture certainly is, early predictions were that the twenty-three pairs of human chromosomes would be packed with a few hundred thousand genes. During the laborious process—aided by laboratory robots but guided by a large group of smart scientists—the narrative morphed from one characterized by hubris to shock and eventually to chagrin. It turns out that we have about half the number of genes as the average potato: around twenty thousand!

The story of this endeavor—bravado, surprise, then humility—is more or less the story of science in general and a microcosm of my personal path. Fortunately, the majority of scientific progress is measured by improvements in the questions we ask rather than the finality of our answers. While many are convinced that cures are just around the corner, it seems to me that the more deeply we look at anything, the more complex and mysterious it becomes. It's as if with each additional data point, our realization of how very little we understand increases proportionately; like an onion with infinite layers. While it is a privilege to be part of this endeavor, after many decades in the field I admit I'm not especially hopeful about the prospects of solving something as complex and intractable as addiction anytime soon. For that matter, I'm increasingly skeptical that the solutions are ever going to be found solely in the brain.

The Queen of Hearts' Solution

There's no lack of conviction that something must be done about the addiction problem. You wouldn't be reading this book if you didn't realize that drug use is a gargantuan crisis. What can be done?

Many of us sympathize with Lewis Carroll's Queen of Hearts who screamed "Off with their heads" in frustration at her subjects' failure to appropriately enact the social order.[2] What else to do with such misbehaving subjects? As a matter of fact, Rodrigo Duterte, the president of the Philippines, adopted something quite like the Queen of Hearts' strategy, with the added efficiency of bullets. Though most of us are appalled by the fact that in just a couple of years emissaries for his war on drugs have killed many thousands of people,[3] we can probably also relate to the frustration that might make Operation Double Barrel seem like the only option. Along similar lines, some U.S. states have considered withholding overdose antidotes like Narcan from repeat offenders, as if letting them die would teach them a lesson.

To lesser degrees, other solutions in the vein of "if you can't control your own behavior, we'll do it for you" are being vetted. In some parts of the world, as we've seen, mesolimbic brain lesions are administered to unwilling addicts, and in the United States we are beginning to offer brain surgery as a possible alternative to prison. To be fair, the deep brain stimulation on offer here may be reversed by turning off the current, but not every strategy proposed would be reversible. For instance, vaccines are being developed that would render a drug of choice moot, and while such antibodies would have narrow effects, they would be permanent. All of these examples have in common a solution aimed at constricting addicts' choices.

As we go down this path, driven by society's desperation to do almost anything to slow the hemorrhage in our families, schools, and towns, there are both practical and ethical issues to consider. For instance, when would interventions like this become viable? Only as a last resort? Solely for those with a bona fide addiction, or perhaps midway through a putative trajectory, before too much damage is done? In that case, why not assess users early in their misuse and intervene to mitigate all harm, before they even have a chance to upend the lives of their families and friends or get a first DUI? Eventually, it might seem advantageous to intervene in children, assessing a combination of genetics, personality traits, teacher reports, and early life experiences to find those with high risk, and prevent disordered use entirely.

Most of us are appalled at such thoughts, because we recognize the many slippery slopes leading from attempts to engineer or control behavior, as well as how much we value our own freedom—even to make mistakes. Some of us might even see our screwups and weaknesses as valuable learning experiences that have helped shape personal strengths. Though we probably wouldn't like or trust some external authority stepping in to prevent or remove the possibility of our errant ways, do we have any viable alternative?

By *any* account, the "war on drugs" has been a recurrent and dismal failure. I would argue that that is because finger-pointing and violence do nothing to subdue the drive to escape the pain of our existence; if anything, they make it worse. In 1917, Congress passed a law that eventually became the Eighteenth Amendment to the U.S. Constitution prohibiting the "manufacture, sale, transportation and importation" of liquor. One of the most robust effects of the prohibition was an increase in illegal manufacture, sale, and transportation of the stuff, and though fewer Americans consumed alcohol during this period, those who did drink, drank more. The amendment was repealed in 1933, widely recognized as a massive failure. Around this same time, Mexican immigrants were being scapegoated for the high unemployment of whites, and because they had also introduced recreational use of marijuana into the United States, the Marijuana Tax Act was passed—as a xenophobic economic initiative rather than anything to do with health. Like laws that followed, little of the drug legislation in this country has been based on scientific evidence of harm. By the end of the twentieth century, despite widespread regulation and stiff penalties, drug use was rampant.

The truth is, people like me who are prone to excessive use are less likely than average to be swayed by outside pressure, including punishment. We're also more likely to ignore public mores—if not to turn against them. When I was growing up, First Lady Nancy Reagan began a campaign to encourage people to "just say no." I've often thought that she might have been more effective had she encouraged experimentation, because many addicts, and certainly I, tend to do the opposite of what they're told.

Efforts aimed at constricting supply only serve to ignite the efforts of those seeking to satisfy their own or others' demand, in the same way that dieters typically gain weight. And this demand is, in many ways, an inevitable part of human nature. Removing the drive to get high, as ancient, ubiquitous, and neurologically relevant as it is, is about as likely to happen as removing our desire to create and explore.

Alternative Ideas

The majority of addicts die as a result of their insane behavior and wreak havoc on the way. But let's be clear: there is nothing exceptional about my recovery; there are millions of happy and successful people who were once as bad off as, or worse off than, I was, and these millions of examples offer a path based in freedom rather than control. Though many, like me, only begin to turn around when we run out of options, ultimately recovery is a process of expansion, not restriction.

I understand firsthand the despair that grows as drugs come to make our choices for us, deciding whom we will be with and what we will do. This gloomy cell of repetition occupied by every addict, despite variation in periodicity, strips us of our most precious commodity, the freedom to choose. This is why I'm not against drugs or drug use, but am so thoroughly opposed to addiction: it strips us of our precious freedom. And this is also why it makes no more sense to cure addiction by imposing permanent or semipermanent limits on our range of choices than it does to teach compassion through corporal punishment. How could one give rise to the other?

Just as children need autonomy in little doses in order to learn restraint, people in recovery obviously can't be entrusted with ourselves all at once. But given social support, a range of attractive alternatives, and perhaps short-term medical interventions, we can learn to choose life—despite its obvious imperfections—over death. Ultimately, this freedom is the antidote to addiction. When I occasionally hear sober people say that using is no longer an option, I cringe. It is precisely an option. That's exactly the point.

So, what might be an ideal cure? First, an easily administered formulation that would obviate withdrawal and craving, removing the biological necessity for a swift relapse. This is important because most daily users can't make it through the first hours of withdrawal without succumbing to an insatiable drive. And this is the easy part of our panacea; it's been done with Suboxone/buprenorphine for opiate addicts, with Chantix/varenicline for smokers, and with benzos for alcoholics, to a lesser degree, because the drug is such a generalist. In each of these cases, the treatment is only effective when coupled with a slow reduction in dose and ample social support (such as Alcoholics or Narcotics Anonymous, which can provide such support for a lifetime). Because stimulant users don't usually crave in the first few days after a binge, it seems as if we should be home free. But as experience has shown, detoxing is only the beginning, and here's where our treatment strategy meets the temptation to take a shortcut. Perpetual medications, deep brain interventions, antibodies, religious dogmas, or congressional edicts are all likely to be counterproductive in the long run. The principle missing in all these formulations is the opportunity for each of us to freely seek a meaningful life.

Hidden Lifts

As a result of sharing needles, I contracted hepatitis C in the 1980s. Though this was not great news, I recognized that I was fortunate not to have acquired HIV/AIDS, which was, and is, being spread in the same way. I lived with the disease for over thirty years before benefiting from the seemingly trivial, though expensive, cure of eighty-four once-a-day pills. I'm thrilled to report that after all this time the virus has been completely eradicated from my body. On the other hand, being clean and sober for more than thirty years hasn't enabled me to "clear" my addiction. I've been able to stay a safe distance from my disease, but don't think for a minute that I've been cured. Of course, the only way to prove that I can't use gracefully would be to self-destruct, like winning a bet that I can't fly by jumping off a building, but I've a strong suspicion based on the nature of my persistent fantasies. For instance, when someone asks, as happens frequently, whether I would like a glass of wine, it's only a few seconds before I realize absolutely not. Why would anyone want just a glass? At the pubs my husband favors, microbrews are listed by their names and alcohol content. Not only do I think that high-content beers are worth more, but I'm secretly disappointed when he picks a low-octane choice and feel he's wasting both time and money. To my way of thinking, the value of any drug is purely in its ability to take me away from myself, and even though I love my life today, I haven't overcome this mind-set.

My disease isn't caused by a virus or a drug, but instead abides in the way my brain responds to pharmacological treats—enthusiastically and profoundly. This tendency and all psychological (and most biological) traits or tendencies are normally distributed in the overall population. Such natural variation is essential for the survival of the species, because changing environments might favor different individuals at different times. As discussed, any risk factor carried by a subset of people is not specific to abusing drugs but confers more general tendencies as well, like a preference for novelty or risk taking, or a willingness to buck the flow. To this day, the surest way to get me to do something is to tell me not to. I'm not proud of my oppositional bias, but it seems to be a core part of my nature; my mother jokes that when I was only two and she told me to "sleep tight," my reply was that I would "sleep loose." Like others with my condition, I also tend to have low harm avoidance, which means that punishment is likely to be even less effective for people like me than it is in the rest of the population. I was probably grounded for half of my early adolescence, but during the rest of the time I made up for it. I was the first among my peers to leap from the barn loft and am still eager today to attempt new things. What is sometimes lauded as "grit" probably contributed to my willingness to go to extreme lengths to score where a more reasonable person would desist. So was I enterprising or exploitative? Persistent or compulsive? Jeopardous or bravely willing to go after what I wanted? I'm sure all these things.

In other words, those with a liability toward addiction in the twenty-first century might also be those most likely to survive and thrive in our distant past, or future. Even today, such factors might be assets for endeavors that benefit from an ability to tolerate—or even seek—uncertainty, or to push on the margins of conventional practice, such as entrepreneurial avocations or scientific research. I'm not saying that one way to be is better, but neither am I saying that it is worse. What's reckless in one context might be innovative in another.

An attitude of latitude in what we value, or even tolerate, couldn't hurt our efforts at a cure. Society, as well as the market, understandably appreciates those among us who are able to toe the line and toss back a few while doing it. But this ability isn't universal, and perhaps we shouldn't try to make it so. Particularly if the way to achieve such a likable ability for moderation is through medication or other invasive strategies.

Context

Another question to consider is the role culture contributes to the disorder. Swings in drug use—like the spike in stimulant abuse coincident with the rise of consumerism in the 1980s that helped take me down, or the present efforts to sleep away the world's suffering—fail to give a true impression of the consistency of the general phenomenon, but they do reflect addiction's context dependency. How I ended up so far away from my self and everything I cared about was undoubtedly part me and part my environment, aided perhaps by poor choices.

On this score, among the most astounding findings in recent neuroscience is the context-dependent nature of all neural activity. Even as our thoughts, feelings, and behaviors are products of neurochemical brain activity, what gives rise to this activity is mostly not in our brains. Rather, our brains express the evolutionary, social, and cultural context we occupy. The brain serves as the dirt from which our thoughts, feelings, and behaviors grow, but these arise as products of substrates within and factors without. We are social creatures, raised in contexts that profoundly influence the structure and activity of our genomes and the electrochemical flow between neurons, and therefore all we do and experience. It follows that the answer to the addiction crisis is not solely in the brain, but must include the context. More than ever before in our evolutionary history, we possess a keen awareness of widespread tragedy and suffering in the world. This is the painful context in which our attempts to avert and deny the burden of consciousness have grown more and more desperate and widespread.

Two important factors are making the situation worse. The first has to do with relatively rapid technological advances in drug potency and delivery. In terms of physiological effects, the difference between chewing on a coca leaf and smoking crack cocaine is like the difference between seeking hydration from a teacup and seeking it from a fire hose. Absorption of cocaine from the leaf is much slower and less efficient than from purified forms of cocaine, so it is literally impossible to achieve the kind of blood concentrations today's addicts readily acquire. In fact, there is no evidence of addiction among people who use coca in its indigenous form. Risk for addiction likewise increased with distillation of alcohol—yielding concentrations way above the limits of fermentation. And so on. As drugs get more potent, they are easier to traffic, and once they are popular, it's a pretty good bet that synthetic versions—with even more potency—are on their way.

Another change in drug use that has been common only for a few hundred years is solitary drug taking as opposed to participating in a culturally endorsed ritual. While surely there were individual cases of excessive drug use in the past, the epidemic incidence of addiction in modern society is dependent on cultural norms that foster, or at least disregard, isolation.

If not a requirement, the tendency to use alone is an index of abuse, as the telescoping of activities and friends toward ensuring the ability to imbibe freely goes hand in hand with developing problems. The obvious reason for this is to avoid people and situations that might question or confront our behavior. Like others, I'd sort activities and relationships based on access to consumables. I would generally avoid interactions that didn't involve getting high but, if I had to participate, would "pregame" to make the exchange more bearable. Friends who didn't support my choice of activities didn't remain friends, and as I progressed in my addiction, I naturally had fewer; the ones I did maintain or develop were those who would collude in the delusion that I was fine (by mirroring my choices). Leigh was a friend-acquaintance who worked with me as a waitress at a burger chain, and I put her in the "friend" category because she liked to party like me. However, after some time away, she returned to work and shared that she'd been to treatment. I can still remember the feeling of shock followed immediately by closing off. I'm not sure if I literally backed away, but I know I'd have been warmer if she'd been diagnosed with an infectious disease! Honestly, this is the last conversation I think we had until I ran into her several years later after getting sober myself. Unfortunately, before we could really reconnect, she overdosed on Dilaudid.

The playing field of our neurobiology is not even, but especially because actions can and do alter our brain's structure and function, we probably have much more influence over the conditions of our lives, and the lives of others, than we realize or utilize. There will always be some of us who are more or less liable to find drugs a handy lever, but we are all positioned somewhere on the same scale. Increased incidence of addiction reflects a tipping of this scale, weighted by the burdens of loneliness; anxiety about the future; isolation despite our Facebook "friends"; the incoherence of institutionalized greed and selfishness; and a social structure that seems to devalue empathy and connection. For example, how does a young adult deal with having to choose between a career that earns a lot of money but depends on exploitation and a career working as one of the exploited? What must it feel like to birth children in a world that doesn't really cherish them? Or to be housed at the end of our days, poor and sick, in warehouses designed just for this purpose? What's really hard to imagine is how anybody wouldn't pick up, faced with realities like these.

And there are plenty who have. Those of us shooting heroin are canaries in the coal mine, desperately trying to escape suffering in the second most direct way imaginable.

So, who's to blame for the epidemic of addiction? The truth is no one is to blame, but we are all responsible. Our collective shadow supports addiction because we must have a scapegoat even as we deny, or embrace, the many strategies of escape we employ ourselves. We support the tools of addiction, including pathological individualism that leads to alienation, widespread and enthusiastic endorsement of avoidance, and a smorgasbord of consumptive excess and self-medication. Though any search for a cause (or a cure) is bound to fall short, one source of this epidemic is our unwillingness to bear our own pain, along with our failure to look upon the suffering of others with compassion. I'm not a masochist, but I do think that pain is underrated as a teacher. My own inevitable failures and weaknesses have been wellsprings for growth and transformation, but only as I face them.

Desperation in any form leads to depraved acts. Social psychology has shown that a primary difference between upstanding citizens and depraved criminals is our circumstances, including many of which are beyond our control. Inherited proclivities, early experiences, and current environments combine to constrain many of our choices. It is not heroin, alcohol, nicotine, or cocaine that makes one an addict; it is the drive to escape from reality. I remember sharing a crack pipe with a homeless man for a while. Though probably only in his early forties, he had few teeth left, and those were dirty and broken. He hadn't showered or even looked in a mirror in weeks and was filthy and emaciated. Yet he'd pull on the pipe and wax on about how he was on top of the world. Even then I was reminded of Huxley's soma, required in some dystopian future in order to cope with society's dementia. Lest we feel above such depravity, we might remember that chemicals aren't the only way to escape. There are plenty of internet and entertainment addicts, food, shopping, or work addicts, maybe as many as there are people who have problems with substances.

The history of every science begins with the individual and progresses to the connected collective. Botany began by cataloging specimens and now understands the health of any species depends on an ecological landscape. Recently botanists are learning that plants communicate with each other—for instance, to warn of insect attack.[4] The focal point for astronomy was earth, thought with certainty to be the center of everything—until Copernicus. Since then, we've realized not only that the earth is a mere speck in the cosmos but that there is no center, only a beginning in the cosmic explosion that is still unfolding under (and around) our feet. In short, now is the time for us to recognize that our brains are not the source of who we are or the path to who we might become.

Humans have a hundred billion neurons in their brains—about as many as there are stars in a galaxy—with an even more astronomical number of synapses through which these cells interact. They are all exquisitely tuned to appreciate and learn from our experiences with each other and the natural world, through connections, communication, our senses, poetry, music, and dance, the world of ideas, and the limits of those ideas. These are the places to turn our attention when hoping to arrest the downward spiral of addiction, because they are considerably more proximal to a cure than anything to be found in another bottle or pill.

Because it could be any of us, because it is many of us, or our loved ones, and because all of us are affected when any fail to realize our full potential, we must commit first of all to acknowledge the problem, to look at it deeply, rather than away from it, and then to reach out to each other with our minds, hearts, and actions, connecting with those who need our help or those whose help we need. To be living on earth today is like being in a lifeboat with every other person on the planet; it's both inhumane and impractical to turn our backs. We are really all in this together. Of course, biology is involved! But the insistence on starting and ending within an addict's head is not only misguided but insidious.

The assistance I speak of is not enabling or excusing. I'm not suggesting we deflect consequences from anyone, not only because it robs them of freedom, but also because it perpetuates the problem. But at the very least, let's acknowledge what we see. As James Baldwin said, "We can't fix what we won't face," so let's see it and say it. Instead of pretending not to notice when mind-altering substances erode our connection to another, either in an uncharacteristic display at the company party or as part of a slowly evolving downward slide, why not share our observations? After being sober for some time, I was stopped at a light early one morning on Spanish River Boulevard in Boca Raton. Glancing over at the car next to me, I noticed a seemingly normal fellow guzzling from a bottle in a brown paper bag. He looked up, and our eyes connected over the edge of the bag. What has haunted me ever since is how thoroughly and quickly I looked away, as if I had done something wrong by noticing his early-morning nip. And I did feel, and can still recollect, a sense of shame and, I'm embarrassed to say, distaste. Why do people who are acting so contrary to their own best interests evoke denial in all of us? A victim of virtually any disease usually elicits pity; addicts mostly evoke revulsion. What is it about the irrational behavior of an addict that makes everyone want to turn away?

Final Words

The opiate epidemic starkly reveals what has been true all along, but perhaps too easy to ignore: most addicts cross over into uncontrolled use in plain sight, without anyone—especially themselves—realizing until it is too late. Once they are across the threshold, their chances of regaining control are vanishingly small. It's striking that despite all neuroscience has learned about addiction, it has had little impact on this path. This is partly because there is still much we don't understand, but mostly because of the incredibly powerful capacity of the brain to thwart drug effects. Though I can certainly appreciate both of these impediments, an even bigger impediment may be the way we respond to each other. Together we nourish the epidemic of addiction by espousing false dichotomies like "us" versus "them" or "well" versus "sick." In doing so, we embrace the myth that happiness can be pursued at the individual level, and therefore perpetuate a culture of isolation and alienation. In so doing, we further preclude the possible benefits that might be realized by a more diverse, inclusive community.

In acknowledging that the problem may not be "in them," we might consider that those struggling with addiction today have enhanced sensitivity to the factors that promote isolation and alienation from themselves and from others and thwart meaningful lives. As a young person, just hearing someone admit that mistakes and suffering are a price of being alive, rather than trying to teach me how to prevent or escape these things, might have helped. It's hard to know for sure, but I wonder if my path might have unfolded differently had I had the chance to face existential questions with the support of wise and empathetic models. As some of my teachers in recovery note, as a society we're suffering from depth deprivation.[5] And depth is found most naturally in honest connections.

At the height of my addiction, when asked about his family, my father would reply that he had two sons. If I made a call to the house and my mother wasn't home when he picked up (these were the days before cells: I'd use a pay phone; he'd answer on a landline), he'd just put the phone back in the cradle. If my mother was home, he wouldn't say a word to me, but she would eventually come on the line. It was simply easier for my father to block the pain of my sad existence from his mind and life. I certainly don't blame him, especially because I was trying to do the same.

Though there were several turning points in my trajectory, it seems profoundly significant that the material change began a few months after the ghost-in-the-mirror episode, when my father inexplicably changed course and took me out for my twenty-third birthday. Federal agents, friends' deaths, expulsions and evictions, physical withdrawal, and myriad other tragedies weren't enough to propel me to change; instead, it was human love and connection. My father's willingness to be seen with me and to treat me with kindness split open my defensive shell of rationalizations and justifications. It broke open the lonely heart that neither of us knew I still had.

Exciting advances in neuroscience are uncovering the biological correlates of addiction. Though there is still much to learn in and out of laboratory settings, we have enough cumulative data to recognize that we/our brains are shaped and constrained by much, much more than our individual biology. And of all these influences, perhaps the most immediate and impactful, and therefore potentially helpful for realizing change, are our connections with each other. We affect each other, including each other's neurobiology, neurochemistry, and behavior, in ways that are direct and profound. As we grapple to respond to the growing population of addicts, we'd do well to recognize that disordered use comes from, thrives in, and creates alienation. This means that building walls to keep us from our emotions or our neighbors will only make things worse, by feeding the epidemic.

When bits of information or data are contextualized, we have knowledge. Knowledge helps us to appreciate what we know and to acknowledge that there is much we don't; together these are the beginnings of understanding. Wisdom grows as understanding births humility and open-mindedness, both requisites for seeing things as they are. In the past hundred years, we've stopped expecting addicts to cure themselves, and that is surely progress. But to wait for a biomedical or any other outside cure is to miss asking questions of ourselves and considering our own role in the epidemic. While we are at it, instead of wringing our hands, we might try reaching for another's.

Acknowledgments

I want to acknowledge all of those who have struggled with substance use, and especially to thank friends in recovery who have shared their experience to guide my way, including many women in Boulder, Portland, Greenville, and Seabrook. I'm particularly grateful to Margaret, Ginny, Sharon, Mary, Nancy, LaVerne, Henrietta, Pam, Lauren, Lindy, and Genelle for encouraging and sustaining me on this adventure of awakening. As I've followed their light, I've also been fed by the courage of Rita, Josie, Fran, Alita, Angela, Fannie, and Anna. I'm grateful, too, to the Wharf Rats and Phellows who've helped me enjoy the ride.

I'm thankful to my parents, brothers, husband, and children, who know my imperfections better than anyone but love me just the same, and particularly to my mother whose faith in goodness has helped to change me, and still does. Martha and David Dolge are family, too: a part of who I am, and who I hope to become.

Of the countless scientists upon whose carefully built boat I ride, I am especially grateful to David Wolgin for introducing me to the joys and frustrations of scientific research, Steven Maier for his generosity and inspiration, and John Crabbe for being simply the most ideal mentor I can imagine. I would be nowhere without each of them. There are many neuroscientists who've helped me succeed by lending their support, and in some cases their laboratory benches, including Nicolas Grahame, Jeffrey Mogil, Joanne Weinberg, Peter Kalivas, and Brian McCool, as well as the many fine scholars at the National Institute on Alcohol Abuse and Alcoholism.

I also benefitted from the instruction of Mrs. Sisolak—a middle school biology instructor who introduced me to studying the natural world—and Gene Gollin at the University of Colorado for emphasizing systems-thinking. Finally, I'm indebted to my Living School teachers Richard, Cynthia, and Jim and fellow students, especially Brent, Ed, Elizabeth, Emma, Fran, Katrina, Lee, Richard, Roy, and Tom who have all helped me connect a head full of curiosity to a life of meaning outside of it.

This book took root in the gracious ground of Volterra, Italy, due largely to the kindness of Marissa Roberto, Stefania del Bufalo, and Giuseppe Ricci. I'm also grateful to Luisa and Elena for their excellent instruction at the Scuola San Lino, and to the children there who befriended my daughter, especially Mariasole, Igor, and Asia, as well as their parents Sylvia and Mario, and Ingrid and Georgio.

Time spent with contemplative communities at Moncks Corner, Gesthemane, and Snowmass was critical to getting ideas on pages, as were the many hours spent at Genelle's cabin on Penns Creek.

I'm indebted to Stephani Allen for sharing her clear vision and efficient action in many times of need, as well as to early readers of the book, especially Bill Rogers, Jane Love, Erin Hahn, Mary Fairbairn, Susan D'Amato, Marty Devereaux, and Deidre O'Connor. These friends and colleagues managed to see something in early drafts that was worth saying, and their encouragement helped me persist. I also want to thank Lena Miskulin, a neuroscience and art double major at Bucknell, for sharing her talent in the drawings that make the book more beautiful.

Still, without the wise and sympathetic agenting of Ellen Geiger, providing just the right balance of encouragement and perspective exactly when I need it, as well as the brilliant assistance of Kristine Puopolo, Daniel Meyer, and the talented team at Doubleday, the book may not have seen the light of day.

Notes

1. BRAIN FOOD

1. Dalton Trumbo, *Johnny Got His Gun* (New York: J. B. Lippincott, 1939).
2. James Olds and Peter Milner, "Positive Reinforcement Produced by Electrical Stimulation of Septal Area and Other Regions of Rat Brain," *Journal of Comparative and Physiological Psychology* 47, no. 6 (1954).
3. Nan Li et al., "Nucleus Accumbens Surgery for Addiction," *World Neurosurgery* 80, no. 3–4 (2013), doi:10.1016/j.wneu.2012.10.007.

2. ADAPTATION

1. Claude Bernard, *Lectures on the Phenomena of Life Common to Animals and Plants,* trans. Hebbel E. Hoff, Roger Guillemin, and Lucienne Guillemin (Springfield, Ill.: Thomas, 1974).
2. Walter B. Cannon, *The Wisdom of the Body* (New York: W. W. Norton, 1932).
3. Richard L. Solomon and John D. Corbit, "An Opponent-Process Theory of Motivation: I. Temporal Dynamics of Affect," *Psychological Review* 81, no. 2 (1974).
4. B. P. Acevedo et al., "Neural Correlates of Long-Term Intense Romantic Love," *Social Cognitive and Affective Neuroscience* 7, no. 2 (2012): 145–59, doi.org/10.1093/scan/nsq092.
5. Macnish's *Anatomy of Drunkenness* was first published in 1827 and was such a hit that many updated editions were published before an expanded version in 1859 that included this observation. Robert Macnish, *The Anatomy of Drunkenness* (Glasgow: W. R. McPhun, 1859).

3. ONE SALIENT EXAMPLE: THC

1. Miles Herkenham et al., "Cannabinoid Receptor Localization in Brain," *Proceedings of the National Academy of Sciences* 87, no. 5 (1990).
2. Downregulation of CB_1 receptors following chronic exposure to drugs that activate THC binding sites has been well established by many studies including, for example, those by Christopher S. Breivogel et al.,

"Chronic Delta9-Tetrahydrocannabinol Treatment Produces a Time-Dependent Loss of Cannabinoid Receptors and Cannabinoid Receptor-Activated G Proteins in Rat Brain," *Journal of Neurochemistry* 73, no. 6 (1999); Laura J. Sim-Selley and Billy R. Martin, "Effect of Chronic Administration of R-(+)-[2,3-Dihydro-5-methyl-3-[(morpholinyl) methyl]pyrrolo[1,2,3-de]-1,4-benzoxazinyl]-(1-naphthalenyl)methanone Mesylate (WIN55,212–2) or Delta(9)-tetrahydrocannabinol on Cannabinoid Receptor Adaptation in Mice," *Journal of Pharmacology and Experimental Therapeutics* 303, no. 1 (2002); João Villares, "Chronic Use of Marijuana Decreases Cannabinoid Receptor Binding and mRNA Expression in the Human Brain," *Neuroscience* 145, no. 1 (2007); Victoria Dalton and Katerina Zavitsanou, "Cannabinoid Effects on CB1 Receptor Density in the Adolescent Brain: An Autoradiographic Study Using the Synthetic Cannabinoid HU210," *Synapse* 64, no. 11 (2010); Jussi Hirvonen et al., "Reversible and Regionally Selective Downregulation of Brain Cannabinoid CB1 Receptors in Chronic Daily Cannabis Smokers," *Molecular Psychiatry* 17, no. 6 (2012).

4. DREAM WEAVERS: OPIATES

1.   David Livingstone, *A Popular Account of Missionary Travels and Researches in South Africa* (London: John Murray, 1861). Shortly after arriving to his first post in Mabotswa in 1844, David Livingstone suffered a lion bite on the shoulder, and subsequently wrote about the experience in his journal. Despite persistent pain from his injury, Livingstone spent most of the rest of his life, about another 30 years, exploring Africa. He was the first European to visit many sites in central, southern, and eastern Africa, and re-named Victoria Falls after his queen, and the island from which he first viewed the falls, in 1855, after himself. I prefer the Bantu Lozi description of the falls and the island, roughly translated as "smoke that thunders" and "place of the rainbow." At any rate, Livingstone dropped out of missionary service because he felt a spiritual calling to political and economic action, hoping to work against slavery by opening up trade routes in Africa. He wasn't especially effective, in part because his expeditions to find new trade routes generally failed. He'd been ill and out of touch for several years by the time the Welsh explorer H. M. Stanley located him in 1871. Livingstone died about a year and a half later of malaria and dysentery at the age of sixty.

2.   Eric Wiertelak, Steven Maier, and Linda Watkins, "Cholecystokinin Antianalgesia: Safety Cues Abolish Morphine Analgesia," *Science* 256, no. 5058 (1992).

5: THE SLEDGEHAMMER: ALCOHOL

1.   Frederick Marryat, *Second Series of a Diary in America, with Remarks on Its Institutions* (Philadelphia: T.K. & P.G. Collins, 1840).

Nicotine," *Annual Review of Neuroscience* 34 (2011), doi:10.1146/annurev-neuro-061010-113734.

7. Aaron Ettenberg, "Opponent Process Properties of Self-Administered Cocaine," *Neuroscience and Biobehavioral Reviews* 27, no. 8 (2004).

8. Juan Sanchez-Ramos, "Neurologic Complications of Psychomotor Stimulant Abuse," in *International Review of Neurobiology: The Neuropsychiatric Complications of Stimulant Abuse,* ed. Pille Taba, Andrew Lees, and Katrin Sikk (Amsterdam: Academic Press, 2015).

9. G. Hatzidimitriou, U. D. McCann, G. A. Ricaurte, "Altered Serotonin Innervation Patterns in the Forebrain of Monkeys Treated with (±)3,4-Methylenedioxymethamphetamine Seven Years Previously: Factors Influencing Abnormal Recovery," *Journal of Neuroscience* 19 (1989): 5096–5107.

10. Lynn Taurah, Chris Chandler, Geoff Sanders, "Depression, Impulsiveness, Sleep, and Memory in Past and Present Polydrug Users of 3,4-Methylene dioxymethamphetamine (MDMA, ecstasy)," *Psychopharmacology* 231 (2014), doi:10.1007/s00213-013-3288-1.

8. SEEING CLEARLY NOW: PSYCHEDELICS

1. Albert Hofmann, "Notes and Documents Concerning the Discovery of LSD," *Agents and Actions* 1, no. 3 (1970), doi.org/10.1007/BFO1986673.

2. "Stanislav Grof Interviews Dr. Albert Hofmann, Esalen Institute, Big Sur, California, 1984," accessed April 14, 2018, www.maps.org.

3. "LSD: The Geek's Wonder Drug?," www.wired.com, Jan. 16, 2006.

4. Diana Kwon, "Trippy Treatments," *Scientist,* Sept. 2017.

5. Michael P. Bogenschutz et al., "Psilocybin-Assisted Treatment for Alcohol Dependence: A Proof-of-Concept Study," *Journal of Psychopharmacology* 29, no. 3 (2015), doi:10.1177/0269881114565144.

6. Peter S. Hendricks et al., "The Relationships of Classic Psychedelic Use with Criminal Behavior in the United States Adult Population," *Journal of Psychopharmacology* 32, no. 1 (2018), doi:10.1177/0269881117735685.

7. R. R. Griffiths et al., "Psilocybin-Occasioned Mystical-Type Experience in Combination With Meditation and Other Spiritual Practices Produces Enduring Positive Changes in Psychological Functioning and in Trait Measures of Prosocial Attitudes and Behaviors," *Journal of Psychopharmacology* 32 (2018): 49–69.

8. José Carlos Bouso et al., "Personality, Psychopathology, Life Attitudes, and Neuropsychological Performance Among Ritual Users of Ayahuasca: A Longitudinal Study," *PLoS ONE* 7, no. 8 (2012), doi.org/10.1371/journal.pone.0042421.

9. Evan J. Kyzar et al., "Psychedelic Drugs in Biomedicine," *Trends in Pharmacological Science* 38, no. 11 (2017).

10. David E. Nichols, Matthew W. Johnson, and Charles D. Nichols, "Psychedelics as Medicines: An Emerging New Paradigm," *Clinical Pharmacology and Therapeutics* 101, no. 2 (2017), doi:10.1002/cpt.557.

9. A WILL AND A WAY: OTHER ABUSED DRUGS

1. Cody J. Wenthur, Bin Zhou, and Kim D. Janda, "Vaccine-Driven Pharmacodynamic Dissection and Mitigation of Fenethylline Psychoactivity," *Nature* 548 (2017), doi:10.1038/nature23464.
2. Xin Wang, Zheng Xu, and Chang-Hong Miao, "Current Clinical Evidence on the Effect of General Anesthesia on Neurodevelopment in Children: An Updated Systematic Review with Meta-regression," *PLoS ONE* 9, no. 1 (2014), doi:10.1371/journal.pone.0085760.
3. Matthew Baggott, E. Erowid, and F. Erowid, "A Survey of *Salvia divinorum* Users," *Erowid Extracts* 6 (June 2004), accessed March 2, 2018.
4. Rachel I. Anderson and Howard C. Becker, "Role of the Dynorphin/ Kappa Opioid Receptor System in the Motivational Effects of Ethanol," *Alcoholism: Clinical and Experimental Research* 41, no. 8 (2017); George F. Koob, "The Dark Side of Emotion: The Addiction Perspective," *European Journal of Pharmacology* 15 (2015).
5. André Cruz et al., "A Unique Natural Selective Kappa-opioid Receptor Agonist, Salvinorin A, and Its Roles in Human Therapeutics," *Phytochemistry* 137 (2017), doi:10.1016/j.phytochem.2017.02.001.
6. Yong Zhang et al., "Effects of the Plant-Derived Hallucinogen Salvinorin A on Basal Dopamine Levels in the Caudate Putamen and in a Conditioned Place Aversion Assay in Mice: Agonist Actions at Kappa Opioid Receptors," *Psychopharmacology* 179, no. 3 (2005); William A. Carlezon Jr. et al., "Depressive-Like Effects of the Kappa-opioid Receptor Agonist Salvinorin A on Behavior and Neurochemistry in Rats," *Journal of Pharmacology and Experimental Therapeutics* 316, no. 1 (2006).
7. Daniela Braida et al., "Involvement of K-opioid and Endocannabinoid System on Salvinorin A–Induced Reward," *Biological Psychiatry* 63, no. 3 (2008).
8. Paul Prather et al., "Synthetic Pot: Not Your Grandfather's Marijuana," *Trends in Pharmacological Sciences* 38, no. 3 (2017), doi:10.1016/j .tips.2016.12.003.
9. David M. Wood, Alan D. Brailsford, and Paul I. Dargan, "Acute Toxicity and Withdrawal Syndromes Related to γ-hydroxybutyrate (GHB) and Its Analogues γ-butyrolactone (GBL) and 1,4-Butanediol (1,4-BD)," *Drug Testing and Analysis* 3, nos. 7–8 (2011), doi:10.1002/dta.292.
10. Matthew O. Howard et al., "Inhalant Use and Inhalant Use Disorders in the United States," *Addiction Science and Clinical Practice* 6, no. 1 (2011).
11. Ibid.
12. Stephen H. Dinwiddie, Theodore Reich, and C. Robert Cloninger, "The Relationship of Solvent Use to Other Substance Use," *American Journal of Drug and Alcohol Abuse* 17, no. 2 (1991).

10. WHY ME?

1. Carl Sagan, "The Burden of Skepticism," *Skeptical Inquirer* 12 (1987).
2. Rachel Yehuda et al., "Holocaust Exposure Induced Intergenerational

Effects on FKBP5 Methylation," *Biological Psychiatry* 80, no. 5 (2016), doi:10.1016/j.biopsych.2015.08.005.

3. Elmar W. Tobi et al., "DNA Methylation Signatures Link Prenatal Famine Exposure to Growth and Metabolism," *Nature Communications* 5 (2014) (erratum in *Nature Communications* 6 [2015]), doi:10.1038/ncomms6592.

4. H. Szutorisz et al., "Parental THC Exposure Leads to Compulsive Heroin-Seeking and Altered Striatal Synaptic Plasticity in the Subsequent Generation," *Neuropsychopharmacology* 39 (2014): 1315–1323.

5. Moshe Szyf, "Nongenetic Inheritance and Transgenerational Epigenetics," *Trends in Molecular Medicine* 21, no. 2 (2015).

6. David M. Fergusson and Joseph M. Boden, "Cannabis Use and Later Life Outcomes," *Addiction* 103, no. 6 (2008); Henrietta Szutorisz et al., "Parental THC Exposure Leads to Compulsive Heroin-Seeking and Altered Striatal Synaptic Plasticity in the Subsequent Generation," *Neuropsychopharmacology* 39, no. 6 (2014), doi.org/10.1038 /npp.2013.352; Eric R. Kandel and Denise B. Kandel, "A Molecular Basis for Nicotine as a Gateway Drug," *New England Journal of Medicine* 371, no. 21 (2014), doi:10.1056/NEJMsa1405092.

7. For a recent review on this topic, see Chloe J. Jordan and Susan L. Andersen, "Sensitive Periods of Substance Abuse: Early Risk for the Transition to Dependence," *Developmental Cognitive Neuroscience* 25 (2017), doi:10.1016/j.dcn.2016.10.004.

8. U.S. Department of Health and Human Services, Office of the Surgeon General, *Facing Addiction in America,* 2016.

9. Rebecca D. Crean, Natania A. Crane, and Barbara J. Mason, "An Evidence Based Review of Acute and Long-Term Effects of Cannabis Use on Executive Cognitive Functions," *Journal of Addictive Medicine* 5, no. 1 (2011), doi:10.1097/ADM.0b013e31820c23fa; F. Markus Leweke and Dagmar Koethe, "Cannabis and Psychiatric Disorders: It Is Not Only Addiction," *Addiction Biology* 13, no. 2 (2008), doi:10.1111/j.1369-1600.2008.00106.x; Daniel T. Malone, Matthew N. Hill, and Tiziana Rubino, "Adolescent Cannabis Use and Psychosis: Epidemiology and Neurodevelopmental Models," *British Journal of Pharmacology* 160, no. 3 (2010), doi:10.1111/j.1476–5381.2010.00721.x; Claudia V. Morris et al., "Molecular Mechanisms of Maternal Cannabis and Cigarette Use on Human Neurodevelopment," *European Journal of Neuroscience* 34, no. 10 (2011), doi:10.1111/j.1460–9568.2011.07884.x.

10. Joshua B. Garfield et al., "Attention to Pleasant Stimuli in Early Adolescence Predicts Alcohol-Related Problems in Mid-adolescence," *Biological Psychology* 108 (May 2015), doi:10.1016/j .biopsycho.2015.03.014.

11. Tali Sharot et al., "Dopamine Enhances Expectation of Pleasure in Humans," *Current Biology* 19, no. 24 (2009), doi.org/10.1016/j .cub.2009.10.025.

12. Dorothy E. Grice et al., "Sexual and Physical Assault History and Posttraumatic Stress Disorder in Substance Dependent Individuals," *American Journal of Addictions* 4, no. 4 (1995); Lisa M. Najavits, Roger D. Weiss, and Sarah R. Shaw, "The Link Between Substance Abuse and

Posttraumatic Stress Disorder in Women: A Research Review," *American Journal of Addictions* 6, no. 4 (1997), doi.org/10.1111/j.1521–0391.1997 .tb00408.x.

13. C. L. Ehlers and I. R. Gizer, "Evidence for a Genetic Component for Substance Dependence in Native Americans," *The American Journal of Psychiatry* 170 (2013): 154–164.

11. SOLVING ADDICTION

1. John C. Eccles, "The Future of the Brain Sciences," in *The Future of the Brain Sciences,* ed. Samuel Bogoch (New York: Plenum Press, 1969).

2. Lewis Carroll, *Alice's Adventures in Wonderland* (London: Macmillan, 1865).

3. Human Rights Watch, *World Report, 2017.*

4. Richard Karban, Louie H. Yang, and Kyle F. Edwards, "Volatile Communication Between Plants That Affects Herbivory: A Meta-analysis," *Ecology Letters* 17, no. 1 (2013); and see Kat McGowan, "The Secret Language of Plants," *Quanta Magazine,* Dec. 16, 2013, www .quantamagazine.org.

5. Center for Action and Contemplation, Albuquerque, N.M., cac.org.

Index